NUTRITION
ACROSS THE LIFESPAN FOR HEALTHY AGING

Proceedings of a Workshop

Leslie Pray, *Rapporteur*

Food Forum

Food and Nutrition Board

Health and Medicine Division

The National Academies of
SCIENCES · ENGINEERING · MEDICINE

THE NATIONAL ACADEMIES PRESS
Washington, DC
www.nap.edu

THE NATIONAL ACADEMIES PRESS 500 Fifth Street, NW Washington, DC 20001

This activity was supported by contracts between the National Academy of Sciences and the National Institutes of Health (HHSN263201200074I); U.S. Department of Agriculture (59-1235-2-114, AG-3A94-P-15-0095, CNPP-IOM-FY-2015-01, and FS_NAS_IOM_FY2015_01); and U.S. Food and Drug Administration (HHSP233201400020B/HHSP23337012), with additional support by Abbott Laboratories, Incorporated; Cargill, Inc.; The Coca-Cola Company; ConAgra Foods; Dr Pepper Snapple Group; General Mills, Inc.; Kellogg Company; Kraft Heinz; Mars, Inc.; Monsanto; Nestlé Nutrition; Ocean Spray Cranberries, Inc.; PepsiCo; and Tate & Lyle. Any opinions, findings, conclusions, or recommendations expressed in this publication do not necessarily reflect the views of any organization or agency that provided support for the project.

International Standard Book Number-13: 978-0-309-45748-4
International Standard Book Number-10: 0-309-45748-3
Digital Object Identifier: https://doi.org/10.17226/24735

Additional copies of this publication are available for sale from the National Academies Press, 500 Fifth Street, NW, Keck 360, Washington, DC 20001; (800) 624-6242 or (202) 334-3313; http://www.nap.edu.

Printed in the United States of America

Suggested citation: National Academies of Sciences, Engineering, and Medicine. 2017. *Nutrition Across the Lifespan for Healthy Aging: Proceedings of a Workshop*. Washington, DC: The National Academies Press. doi: https://doi.org/10.17226/24735.

The National Academies of

SCIENCES • ENGINEERING • MEDICINE

The **National Academy of Sciences** was established in 1863 by an Act of Congress, signed by President Lincoln, as a private, nongovernmental institution to advise the nation on issues related to science and technology. Members are elected by their peers for outstanding contributions to research. Dr. Marcia McNutt is president.

The **National Academy of Engineering** was established in 1964 under the charter of the National Academy of Sciences to bring the practices of engineering to advising the nation. Members are elected by their peers for extraordinary contributions to engineering. Dr. C. D. Mote, Jr., is president.

The **National Academy of Medicine** (formerly the Institute of Medicine) was established in 1970 under the charter of the National Academy of Sciences to advise the nation on medical and health issues. Members are elected by their peers for distinguished contributions to medicine and health. Dr. Victor J. Dzau is president.

The three Academies work together as the **National Academies of Sciences, Engineering, and Medicine** to provide independent, objective analysis and advice to the nation and conduct other activities to solve complex problems and inform public policy decisions. The National Academies also encourage education and research, recognize outstanding contributions to knowledge, and increase public understanding in matters of science, engineering, and medicine.

Learn more about the National Academies of Sciences, Engineering, and Medicine at **www.national-academies.org**.

PLANNING COMMITTEE FOR A WORKSHOP ON NUTRITION ACROSS THE LIFESPAN[1]

PAMELA STARKE-REED (*Chair*), Deputy Administrator, Nutrition, Food Safety and Quality, Agricultural Research Service, U.S. Department of Agriculture, Beltsville, Maryland

JOHANNA DWYER, Senior Nutrition Scientist, Office of Dietary Supplements, National Institutes of Health; Director, Frances Stern Nutrition Center, Tufts-New England Medical Center; Professor, Tufts University Medical School and Friedman School of Nutrition Science and Policy, Tufts University, Boston, Massachusetts

GORDON L. JENSEN, Senior Associate Dean for Research, Professor of Medicine and Nutrition, The University of Vermont Larner College of Medicine, Burlington

CATHERINE KWIK-URIBE, Global Director, Health and Nutrition, Mars, Inc., Germantown, Maryland

SHARON A. ROSS, Program Director, Nutritional Science Research Group, Division of Cancer Prevention, National Cancer Institute, National Institutes of Health, Rockville, Maryland

MARY T. STORY, Professor of Global Health and Community and Family Medicine, Associate Director, Education and Training, Duke Global Health Institute, Duke University, Durham, North Carolina

REGINA L. TAN, Director, Office of Food Safety, Food and Nutrition Service, U.S. Department of Agriculture, Alexandria, Virginia

CONNIE WEAVER, Distinguished Professor and Department Head, Department of Nutrition Science, Purdue University, West Lafayette, Indiana

[1]The National Academies of Sciences, Engineering, and Medicine's planning committees are solely responsible for organizing the workshop, identifying topics, and choosing speakers. The responsibility for the published Proceedings of a Workshop rests with the workshop rapporteur and the institution.

FOOD FORUM[1]

SYLVIA ROWE (*Chair*), SR Strategy, LLC, Washington, DC
ARTI ARORA, The Coca-Cola Company, Atlanta, Georgia
CONNIE AVRAMIS, Unilever Research and Development, Englewood Cliffs, New Jersey
FRANCIS (FRANK) BUSTA, University of Minnesota, St. Paul
PAUL M. COATES, Office of Dietary Supplements, National Institutes of Health, Bethesda, Maryland
DAVID B. COCKRAM, Abbott Laboratories, Incorporated, Columbus, Ohio (*through December 2016*)
NAOMI FUKAGAWA, Agricultural Research Service, U.S. Department of Agriculture, Beltsville, Maryland
DAVID GOLDMAN, Food Safety and Inspection Service, U.S. Department of Agriculture, Washington, DC
DANIEL A. GOLDSTEIN, Monsanto, St. Louis, Missouri
DANIELLE GREENBURG, PepsiCo, Purchase, New York
SONYA A. GRIER, American University, Washington, DC
JEAN HALLORAN, Consumers Union, Yonkers, New York
JACKIE HAVEN, Center for Nutrition Policy and Promotion, U.S. Department of Agriculture, Alexandria, Virginia
KATE J. HOUSTON, Cargill Inc., Washington, DC
LEE-ANN JAYKUS, North Carolina State University, Raleigh
GORDON L. JENSEN, Pennsylvania State University, University Park (*through December 2016*)
HELEN H. JENSEN, Iowa State University, Ames
RENÉE S. JOHNSON, Library of Congress, Washington, DC
WENDY L. JOHNSON-ASKEW, Gerber Products Company, Florham Park, New Jersey
CHRISTINA KHOO, Ocean Spray Cranberries, Inc., Lakeville, Massachusetts
VIVICA KRAAK, Virginia Tech, Blacksburg
SUSAN M. KREBS-SMITH, Division of Cancer Control and Population Sciences, National Cancer Institute, National Institutes of Health, Bethesda, Maryland
CATHERINE KWIK-URIBE, Mars, Inc., Germantown, Maryland
CHRISTOPHER JOHN LYNCH, National Institute of Diabetes and Digestive and Kidney Diseases, National Institutes of Health, Bethesda, Maryland

[1]The National Academies of Sciences, Engineering, and Medicine's forums and roundtables do not issue, review, or approve individual documents. The responsibility for the published Proceedings of a Workshop rests with the workshop rapporteur and the institution.

SUSAN MAYNE, U.S. Food and Drug Administration, College Park, Maryland
KAREN McINTYRE, Health Canada, Ottawa, Ontario, Canada
S. SUZANNE NIELSEN, Purdue University, West Lafayette, Indiana
ERIK D. OLSON, Natural Resources Defense Council, Washington, DC
ROBERT POST, Chobani, LLC, New York, New York
KRISTIN REIMERS, ConAgra Foods, Omaha, Nebraska
CLAUDIA RIEDT, Dr Pepper Snapple Group, Plano, Texas
SARAH ROLLER, Kelley Drye & Warren LLP, Washington, DC
SHARON A. ROSS, Division of Cancer Prevention, National Cancer Institute, National Institutes of Health, Bethesda, Maryland
JACQUELINE SCHULZ, The Kraft Heinz Company, Northfield, Illinois (*through December 2016*)
LISA SPENCE, Tate & Lyle, Hoffman Estates, Illinois
PAMELA STARKE-REED, Agricultural Research Service, U.S. Department of Agriculture, Beltsville, Maryland
MAHA TAHIRI, General Mills, Inc., Minneapolis, Minnesota
REGINA TAN, Office of Food Safety, Food and Nutrition Service, U.S. Department of Agriculture

Health and Medicine Division Staff

HEATHER DEL VALLE COOK, Co-Director
LESLIE J. SIM, Co-Director
ANNA BURY, Research Assistant
GERALDINE KENNEDO, Administrative Assistant
ANN YAKTINE, Director, Food and Nutrition Board

Reviewers

This Proceedings of a Workshop has been reviewed in draft form by individuals chosen for their diverse perspectives and technical expertise. The purpose of this independent review is to provide candid and critical comments that will assist the institution in making its published Proceedings of a Workshop as sound as possible and to ensure that the Proceedings of a Workshop meets institutional standards for objectivity, evidence, and responsiveness to the study charge. The review comments and draft manuscript remain confidential to protect the integrity of the process. We wish to thank the following individuals for their review of this Proceedings of a Workshop:

LAWRENCE J. APPEL, Johns Hopkins Medical Institutions, Baltimore, Maryland
DANIEL BELSKY, Duke University, Durham, North Carolina
KRISTA SCOTT, Childcare Aware of America, Arlington, Virginia
PAMELA STARKE-REED, Agricultural Research Service, U.S. Department of Agriculture, Beltsville, Maryland

Although the reviewers listed above provided many constructive comments and suggestions, they did not see the final draft of the Proceedings of a Workshop before its release. The review of this Proceedings of a Workshop was overseen by **JAMES M. NTAMBI,** University of Wisconsin–Madison. He was responsible for making certain that an independent examination of this Proceedings of a Workshop was carried out in accordance with institutional procedures and that all review comments were carefully considered. Responsibility for the final content of this Proceedings of a Workshop rests entirely with the rapporteur and the institution.

Contents

Box and Figures

BOX

FIGURES

1

Introduction

On September 13-14, 2016, a planning committee for the Food Forum of the National Academies of Sciences, Engineering, and Medicine[1] convened a workshop in Washington, DC, to (1) examine trends and patterns in aging and factors related to healthy aging in the United States, with a focus on nutrition; (2) examine how nutrition can sustain and promote healthy aging, not just in late adulthood, but beginning in pregnancy and early childhood and extending throughout the lifespan; (3) highlight the role of nutrition in the aging process at various stages in life; (4) discuss changes in organ systems, including the skeletal, muscular, and cardiovascular systems, over the lifespan, and changes that occur with age related to cognitive, brain, and mental health and to diet-related sensory preferences, oral health, and the microbiome; and (5) explore opportunities to move forward in promoting healthy aging in the United States. See Box 1-1 for the full statement of task for the workshop.

It is important to note that this Proceedings of a Workshop summarizes information presented and discussed at the workshop and is not intended to serve as a comprehensive overview of the subject. Nor are the citations herein intended to serve as a comprehensive set of references for any topic;

[1]The planning committee's role was limited to planning the workshop. This Proceedings of a Workshop was prepared by the rapporteur as a factual account of what occurred at the workshop. Statements, recommendations, and opinions expressed are those of individual presenters and participants and have not been endorsed or verified by the National Academies of Sciences, Engineering, and Medicine. They should not be construed as reflecting any group consensus.

BOX 1-1
Statement of Task

An ad hoc committee will plan and conduct a 2-day public workshop that will explore the current state of knowledge regarding the role of communications and marketing on consumer knowledge and behavior, specifically related to how commercial and public health messaging concerning food, nutrition, and food safety inform, influence, and impact the population at the individual, family, and community levels regarding food choices and behavior.

The workshop agenda will include presentations and discussion that will address scientific credibility, the role of scientific communications in consumer knowledge and behavior related to food and nutrition, and the impact of marketing on consumer decision making. The committee will develop the workshop agenda, select and invite speakers and discussants, and moderate the discussions. After the workshop, a brief workshop summary and full workshop summary of the event will be prepared by a designated rapporteur in accordance with institutional guidelines.

only references cited on speaker slides or in the workshop briefing notebook are included.

The organization of this Proceedings of a Workshop parallels the organization of the workshop (see Appendix A for the workshop agenda). Chapter 2, "Changing Landscape: Demographics, Health Status, and Nutritional Needs," summarizes the Session 1 presentations and discussion. Speakers provided an overview of the demographics, health status, and nutritional needs of the older U.S. population. Chapter 3, "The Spectrum of Aging and Health Over the Lifespan," summarizes the Session 2 presentations and discussion, with a focus on aging over the lifespan (e.g., how risk factors early in life predict health outcomes later in life). Chapter 4, "Changes in Organ Systems Over the Lifespan," summarizes the Session 3 presentations and discussion. Speakers covered a range of organ systems, including the cardiovascular system, skeletal and muscular systems, sensory and oral health, and the gut and gut microbiome. Chapter 5, "Moving Forward," summarizes the Session 4 presentations and discussion, in which the focus of the workshop shifted to the future and ways to promote healthy aging. Finally, Chapter 6, "Healthy Aging: What Is It? Are There Acceptable Markers to Utilize in Developing Strategies to Promote It?," is a summary of the workshop's closing moderated discussion.

2

Changing Landscape: Demographics, Health Status, and Nutritional Needs

In the opening session, moderated by Pamela Starke-Reed, deputy administrator for nutrition, food safety, and quality, Agricultural Research Service, U.S. Department of Agriculture, speakers provided an overview of the demographics, health status, and nutritional needs of the older U.S. population.

Drawing on the most recent report issued by the Federal Interagency Forum on Aging-related Statistics—*Older Americans 2016: Key Indicators of Well-Being* (Federal Interagency Forum on Aging-related Statistics, 2016), which itself draws on multiple data sources—Jennifer Madans, associate director for science, National Center for Health Statistics, described trends in six categories of key indicators of well-being in the U.S. population of older adults. Mary Ann Johnson, Bill and Jane Flatt professor in foods and nutrition, College of Family and Consumer Sciences, and interim director, Institute of Gerontology, College of Public Health, University of Georgia, then discussed healthy aging as not only living a long life but also living in good health, and reviewed several different methodological approaches researchers have been using to identify biomarkers of healthy aging.

THE CHANGING FACE OF OLDER AMERICANS: KEY INDICATORS OF WELL-BEING[1]

Drawing exclusively on the most recent report of the Federal Interagency Forum on Aging-related Statistics (2016)—*Older Americans 2016:*

[1]This section summarizes information presented by Dr. Madans.

Key Indicators of Well-Being—Madans described trends in the following six categories of key indicators of well-being in the older U.S. population: population characteristics, economic indicators, health status, health risks and behavior, health care, and environmental indicators.

The Federal Interagency Forum on Aging-related Statistics, Madans explained, was established in 1986 by the National Institute on Aging of the National Institutes of Health in cooperation with the National Center for Health Statistics and the U.S. Census Bureau. Today it includes 16 federal agencies. The group was formed, Madans explained, to foster collaboration among federal agencies that either produce or use statistical data on the older population, to improve cooperation across agencies and disciplines, and to improve consistency in how data on the aging population are reported. One way for the forum to carry out its mission, she said, is to compile periodic reports on indicators of well-being for this population from across the federal data system. Madans noted that although these reports are issued every 3-4 years, the data tables are updated online more frequently. The report covers 41 indicators in the six categories cited above. Additionally, every report also has a special feature. The special feature in the 2016 report is on informal caregiving.

Madans explained that the indicators she would be presenting were among those that are related to nutrition; moreover, because the report itself draws on multiple data sources, some of the data cover the entire U.S. population, while other data cover only the civilian noninstitutionalized (i.e., household) population. She emphasized that the report contains a wealth of information on the well-being of older Americans that could not be covered in her brief presentation.

Population Characteristics

Madans reported that the number of people in the United States aged 65 and over increased from about 3 million in 1900 to about 46 million in 2014. She highlighted the especially large increase in the number of people in this age group in 2011, which is when the baby boomers (those born after the end of World War II, between 1946 and 1964) began turning 65 (see Figure 2-1). This large increase in the number of people aged 65 and over is expected to continue, she observed, but the growth rate is projected to slow after 2030, when the last of the baby boomers turn 65. Although the numbers of people in this age group will continue to increase, she remarked that they will plateau as a percentage of the total U.S. population at around 21 percent sometime between 2020 and 2030. The population aged 85 and over is projected to see rapid growth after 2030 as the baby boomers enter this age range. Compared with about 100,000 in 1900, Madans noted, an

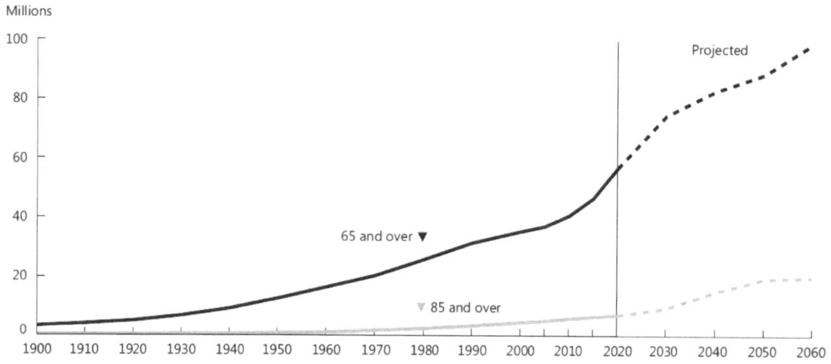

FIGURE 2-1 Population aged 65 and over and aged 85 and over, selected years, 1900-2014, and projected years, 2020-2060.
SOURCES: Presented by J. Madans, September 13, 2016. From Federal Interagency Forum on Aging-related Statistics, 2016.

expected 20 million people over age 85 will be living in the United States by 2060 according to projections.

Madans explained that the future projections illustrated in Figure 2-1—for example, that 90 million people aged 65 and older are projected out to 2060—are a function of assumptions about mortality rates. She noted that these assumptions are more accurate for the near than for the more distant future.

Not only are the numbers of people aged 65 and 85 and older increasing, Madans continued, but the demographic characteristics of these populations are also changing. She highlighted education first, she said, because it is related to so many other factors, such as income, as well as to lifestyle characteristics that affect nutrition. The percentages of the U.S. population aged 65 and older with a high school diploma and with a bachelor's degree have been increasing since 1965 (see Figure 2-2). By 2015, 84 percent of the U.S. population had at least a high school education, and 27 percent had a bachelor's degree or higher.

In addition to educational attainment, Madans continued, living arrangements can have major effects on people's lives. She showed data on living arrangement for 2015 by both sex and race/ethnicity. She remarked that people sometimes think of the 65 and older population "monolithically," as though they were all the same, but, she said, "That is certainly not true." She argued that examining indicators by sex and by race/ethnicity provides insight into this population's heterogeneity. Most individuals aged

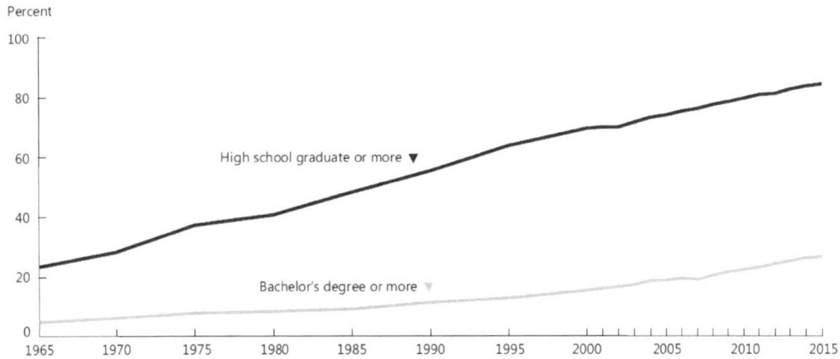

FIGURE 2-2 Educational attainment of the U.S. population aged 65 and older, selected years, 1965-2015.
SOURCES: Presented by J. Madans, September 13, 2016. From Federal Interagency Forum on Aging-related Statistics, 2016.

65 and older still live in the community, she said. The majority, especially among men, are living with a spouse, with implications for shopping, eating (nutrition), and health care. Madans reported that among those aged 65 and older, 45 percent of women are living with a spouse, compared with 70 percent of men; women are more likely to live alone (36 percent) or with other relatives (16 percent) compared with men (20 percent and 6 percent, respectively). She emphasized the variation by race and ethnicity in these characteristics. Among black women, for example, compared with other racial/ethnic groups, higher percentages live alone (43 percent) or with other relatives (30 percent), and a lower percentage live with a spouse (24 percent). Similarly for black men, a higher percentage live alone (30 percent, compared with 20 percent across all racial/ethnic groups).

Economic Indicators

Madans reported that since 1974 there has been a relatively large increase in the percentage of the population aged 65 and over living at 400 percent or greater above the federal poverty threshold. In 2014, she noted, 36 percent of the 65 and over population was in this higher income group. Meanwhile, she said, the percentage of people 65 and over living in poverty has declined, to about 10 percent in 2014. The percentage living at 100 to 199 percent above the poverty threshold has declined as well, to 23 percent in 2014. In 2014, 31 percent of the population 65 and older was living at between 200 and 399 percent above the poverty threshold. This overall improvement in the income distribution among this older population is due to many factors, Madans said, including education and changes in public policies.

With respect to sources of income, Madans continued, overall, 86 percent of this population in 2014 lived in families with income from social security, 59 percent were receiving income from pensions, and 67 percent were receiving some income from assets. More specifically, she noted, income from social security accounted for 49 percent of family income, income from earnings for 24 percent, and pensions for 16 percent. She observed that the percentage distribution of per capita income for those 65 and older varies across income quintiles (i.e., lowest through highest fifth). In the lowest quintile, she said, social security is a much greater sole source of income (67 percent of people in this age group) relative to the highest quintile (18 percent). She went on to report that, relative to the lowest quintile, those in the highest quintile receive much more of their income only from earnings (40 percent) or pensions (26 percent).

With respect to how this money is spent, Madans said, housing continues to be the largest expenditure, as it is among those aged 55-64, accounting for 32 to 37 percent of income among individuals aged 65 and older. She finds it interesting that the amount spent on food does not change much with age, accounting for 13 percent of income among those aged 65 and older, compared with 12 percent among those aged 55-64. She went on to note that health care expenditures show a slight increase, from 9 percent among those 55-64 to 12 percent among those 65-74 and 16 percent among those 75 and older.

Health Status

Madans noted that health status indicators include life expectancy, which since 1981 and at both ages 65 and 85 has increased for both women and men and among both the white and black populations. Additionally, she pointed out, variation in life expectancy among these groups (at both ages 65 and 85) has declined over time (i.e., since 1981). Today (based on 2014 data), life expectancy at age 65 is higher for the white than for the black population, but that differential, which is about 3.4 years at birth, drops to 1.1 years at age 65 and then switches at age 85, with the black population having a higher life expectancy of about half a year. It has been suggested, Madans noted, that this pattern may reflect in part the fact that death rates in the black population are higher in the younger age groups, so that the surviving cohort may be more robust. There have also been some issues with misreporting of age, she observed, particularly on death certificates, on which, mainly in the past, age tended to be overestimated.

Regarding the sex differential in life expectancies, women continue to have longer life expectancies than men at birth at both ages 65 and 85.

Another health status indicator, Madans continued, is cause of death. Since 1981, there has been a major decline in death rates due to heart disease among individuals 65 and older. In fact, she remarked, death rates have declined for all leading causes of death except Alzheimer's disease and unintended injuries. She commented that many people are watching the death rate trajectories for heart disease and cancer, wondering whether and when cancer will become the leading cause of death. Although this has not yet happened nationally, she noted that it has happened in some states and among some age groups. In her opinion, the greater issue of concern with respect to cause of death is that most mortality statistics are based on underlying cause of death. This is an issue, she explained, because there can be only one underlying cause of death per death certificate, yet it can be very difficult to disentangle the underlying cause of death (i.e., the cause that set in motion the process that ultimately led to death) from the other, often multiple, causes listed on the certificate. The number of chronic conditions increases with age, she noted, so more conditions contribute to death. Moreover, she emphasized, there is a difference between dying *from* a disease and dying *with* that disease. This is particularly an issue for Alzheimer's disease death rates, she remarked, when Alzheimer's may not be the underlying cause of death but have contributed to the death or when it may be present but not related to the death. The same is true of diabetes, she said. In her opinion, more information about mortality in the older population can be obtained from examining multiple causes of death, although doing so creates a statistical challenge because of double counting. She believes these issues should be considered in evaluating mortality statistics based on underlying causes of death in populations with multiple chronic conditions.

The most prevalent chronic health conditions in the noninstitutionalized population aged 65 and older are similar to the leading causes of death, Madans observed. In addition to heart disease and hypertension, however, this population experiences high rates of arthritis, which, although it does not affect death, does affect functioning.

Older Americans 2016 provides information on three oral health indicators: dental insurance, dental visits per year, and natural teeth. Dental insurance decreases with age, Madans noted, with 30 percent of people aged 65-74 and over carrying this insurance compared with 20 percent of those aged 75-84 and 16 percent of those aged 85 and over. Dental visits in the past year decline as well, she reported, from 66 percent of people aged 65-74 to 58 percent of those aged 75-84 and 56 percent of those aged 85 and over. The percentage of people with no natural teeth rises from 16 percent of people aged 65-74 to 25 percent of those aged 75-84 and 31 percent of those aged 85 and over.

Dementia is a major health issue for this age group, Madans continued. Data on dementia in *Older Americans 2016* are based on a combination of diagnosed dementia and cognitive testing, she noted. The percentage of the non-nursing home population aged 65 and over with dementia increases with age among both men and women, she observed: 5 percent and 3 percent, respectively, for those aged 65-74; 11 percent and 13 percent, respectively, for those aged 75-84; and 24 percent and 30 percent, respectively, for those 85 and over.

Looking a little more broadly at functional limitations in general (i.e., including limitations in vision, hearing, mobility, communication, cognition, and self-care), Madans reported that in 2014, 19 percent of men and 24 percent of women aged 65 and over had any of these limitations. Of the specific functional limitations included in this indicator, mobility limitations are the most prevalent, she said, affecting 11 percent of men and 17 percent of women in this age group.

Health Risks and Behavior

In the category of health risks and behavior, Madans observed that the quality of the diet of older Americans does not meet recommended standards, especially with respect to sodium; only whole fruit and total protein Healthy Eating Index (HEI)-2010 scores were at or close to 100 (i.e., the standard), which reflects an average diet. The same is true of physical activity, she reported. Although some increase has been seen over time (i.e., since 1998) with respect to the percentage of people aged 65 and older meeting the 2008 federal guidelines for physical activity, still only 12 percent met these guidelines in 2014. Finally, obesity rates among older adults have been increasing since the 1980s, with rates being higher among the younger old (i.e., aged 65 to 74) than among the older old (i.e., 75 and older). In 2011-2014, about 40 percent of people aged 65-74 and about 30 percent of those aged 75 and older had obesity.

Health Care

Health care expenditure data indicate large age differences in spending on health care over time, Madsen reported, with people aged 85 and older spending the most but with the differences between the older age groups becoming smaller over time (i.e., from 1992 to 2012). Annual health care costs for those 85 and older decreased between 1992 and 2012, she noted, compared with a slight increase among younger old-age groups (i.e., 65-74 and 75-84). Most of these expenditures are going to physician and outpatient care, she observed, a consistent trend from 2008 through 2012.

In terms of residential services being provided to the 65 and older population, Madans reiterated that most of this population is living in the community. Among those 85 and older, she reported, 77 percent are living in the community, 15 percent in long-term care facilities, and 8 percent in community housing with services (e.g., meal preparation, transportation, housekeeping).

Looking more broadly at providers of long-term care, Madans noted that most users of such care are receiving home care (i.e., care provided by home health agencies). Home health care is distributed fairly equally among the different old-age categories (i.e., 65-74, 75-84, and 85 and older), she said, but a greater percentage of those 85 and older relative to those 65-74 and 75-84 are receiving care in nursing homes and hospices.

Environmental Indicators

Finally, with respect to environmental indicators of well-being in the older population, Madans focused on how time is used. Across all older age categories, the largest percentage of the day is spent sleeping. Madans noted that this percentage increases slightly with age from 35 percent among people 55-64, to 37 percent among those 65-74, and 38 percent among those 75 and over.

Also with age, Madans added, people spend more time engaged in leisure activities, which account for 33 percent of time among people 75 and older, compared with 29 percent among those 65-74 and 23 percent among those 55-64. Most leisure time is spent watching television, which represents 56 percent of leisure time among people 75 and over, compared with 58 percent and 60 percent among people 65-74 and 55-64, respectively. Madans suggested that what people eat while they watch television may explain many of the trends she had described.

Finally, Madans reported that leisure time spent socializing and communicating decreases with age, from 11 percent of leisure time among those 55-64 and 65-74 to 9 percent among those 75 and older, while time spent reading increases, from 7 percent and 9 percent in the 55-64 and 65-74 age groups, respectively, to 14 percent among those 75 and older. Generally, she observed, solitary leisure time increases with age.

HEALTHY AGING PERSPECTIVE[2]

Johnson began by asking, "What is health?" The World Health Organization (WHO) defines health as "a state of complete physical, mental, and social well-being and not merely the absence of disease or infirmity" (WHO, 1948). Johnson asserted that nutritionists usually think about health from the physical perspective, but that the concept is much broader than this.

What Is Healthy Aging?

Next, Johnson asked, "What is healthy aging?" She described it as not only living a long life but also living in good health. Living a long life, she said, is a result of interactions between genes and the environment, including the nutritional environment. Over the course of the lives of many people living today, she said, living conditions have improved. This improvement, she observed, has resulted in decreased mortality, relaxed evolutionary pressures for early survival and reproduction, greater resource investment in body maintenance and repair, and increased average life expectancies and maximum lifespans (Westendorp, 2006). Healthy aging involves not only reductions in mortality, she argued, but also reductions in morbidity, including chronic conditions, mobility limitations, limitations in activities of daily living (i.e., eating, bathing, dressing, toileting, transferring/walking, continence), sensory changes, and declining cognition.

Johnson continued by stating that population-level metrics of healthy aging include both life expectancy and healthy life expectancy. She defined the latter as life expectancy minus years lived in less than full health as a result of disease and/or injury. In 2013, she noted, average life expectancy across the Americas at birth was 77 years, but average healthy life expectancy was only 67 years (UN, 2015). Another way to look at healthy life expectancy, she said, is to focus on age 65 (as opposed to at birth). In the United States, she reported, healthy life expectancy at age 65 varies among states (see Figure 2-3), from 80 or greater (i.e., an additional 15 years or more) in some states to less than 78 (i.e., fewer than 13 more years) in others (CDC, 2013). She asserted that this variation reflects significant health disparities, particularly in the southern region of the United States.

Biomarkers of Healthy Aging

Johnson said she used to think that biomarkers were things that could be measured only in the blood. But in older adults, she said, biomarkers

[2]This section summarizes information presented by Dr. Johnson.

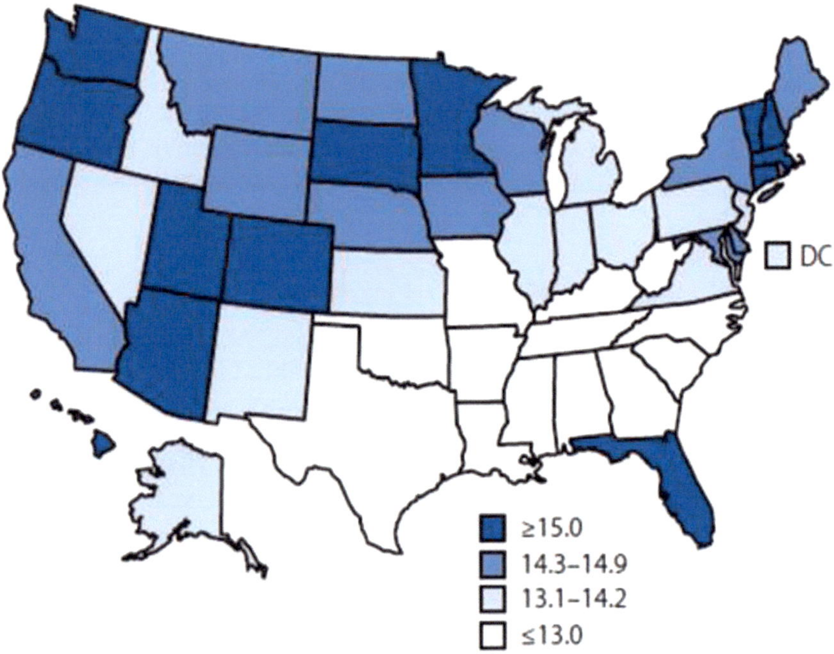

FIGURE 2-3 State-specific healthy life expectancy at age 65, 2007-2009.
NOTE: Healthy life expectancy is calculated from a combination of mortality data and morbidity or health status data.
SOURCES: Presented by M. A. Johnson, September 13, 2016. From CDC, 2013.

are about "so much more." Biomarkers of healthy aging, she noted, include markers of disease onset, progression, and severity; physiological function; endocrine and immune function; and inflammatory responses. They also include genetic markers. But what becomes increasingly important as people age, Johnson asserted, both for older adults themselves and for the people who care for them, is physical and mental capability, including concerns about averting cognitive decline and Alzheimer's disease, maintaining independence (e.g., being able to live in one's own home and do things by oneself), avoiding nursing home admissions, and preventing hospital readmissions.

Johnson provided several examples of different ways in which investigators search for biomarkers of healthy aging. In her opinion, it is important to consider the rationale behind the different biomarkers when thinking about which biomarker to use in designing a new food, for example, or studying a disease or care process.

First, Johnson explained, are aging rates used in cellular and animal studies, which show that the expression of age-related diseases begins in midage and that changing the diet by reducing calories, reducing protein, or balancing micronutrients can delay this expression and lead to healthy aging and longevity (Dato et al., 2016). However, she cautioned against directly translating results from cellular and animal studies to humans, as Dato and colleagues (2016) also caution. With respect to reducing protein, for example, she remarked that the human protein requirement may be higher than current recommended levels. With respect to caloric restriction, she continued, there is a high level of food insecurity in populations with the highest chronic disease incidence, prevalence, and severity.

Next are biologic age biomarkers being examined in the MARK-AGE study, a large, collaborative study across Europe that has recruited more than 3,000 people aged 35-74 (Bürkle et al., 2015). In most such studies, Johnson said, learning something unique about the oldest group of people requires understanding what is going on in younger age groups as well. In addition to recruiting across a wide age range, she explained, the researchers are selecting people from long-lived families, such as 90-year-old sibling pairs, and some of the participants will also undergo a longitudinal phase of the study. Finally, she noted, the researchers have recruited a small number of participants with aging-related genetic disorders, such as progeria (accelerated aging).

Johnson described some of the work behind the MARK-AGE study, beginning with recruitment (i.e., figuring out how to recruit). She reported that the researchers are collecting data on a number of markers, including DNA-based markers, markers based on proteins and their modifications, immunological markers, clinical chemistry markers, hormones, markers of metabolism, and oxidative stress markers. She noted that such a massive amount of data has required addressing data analysis and bioinformatics challenges. Finally, she said, the researchers have been challenged by the many ethical issues that come with knowing so much about so many people. She suggested that as the data become available, this will be a "study to watch."

Another approach to identifying healthy aging biomarkers, Johnson continued, involved developing a longevity phenotype and creating what is called a Healthy Aging Index (Sanders et al., 2014). Here, she said, rather than generating a large set of potential biomarkers, the researchers wanted to identify a subset of markers that are very good predictors of mortality and are heritable. The data examined for this study came from the Cardiovascular Health Study, an ongoing study of risk for cardiovascular disease in about 6,000 participants aged 65 and older. Through a series of analyses, Johnson explained, the researchers identified five indicators of mortality: (1) systolic blood pressure, (2) pulmonary vital capacity, (3) serum creatinine (for kidney function), (4) fasting glucose, and (5) cognitive function (based on the modified Mini-Mental Status Examination). They combined these five indicators by assigning each a score of 0, 1, or 2 based on clinical cutoff, with a maximum Healthy Aging Index score of 10 for an individual. When they compared the worst- and best-tertile scores, the mortality hazard ratio was 2.62. Johnson suggested, that given how predictive of decreased mortality the above five biomarkers were, one way to study how nutrition impacts mortality would be to see how it impacts these biomarkers.

Reflecting on the heritable nature of the biomarkers identified by Sanders and colleagues (2014), which the researchers analyzed in a separate study, Johnson highlighted the importance of being mindful of the genetic underpinning of any biomarker for healthy aging. "Nutrition can do a lot," she said, "but it's going to be working in concert with our genetics."

There have been so many studies of mortality predictors, Johnson continued, that it now is possible to conduct systematic reviews of these studies. She highlighted a review of 23 cohort studies that met the researchers' inclusion criteria (Barron et al., 2015)—that the predictors be blood markers (because of their noninvasive nature) and that the baseline sample age be between 50 and 75 (which is how Barron and colleagues [2015] define midage). Among these 23 studies, she observed, the researchers found 51 potential biomarkers. Of these, they identified 20 actual biomarkers, including 25-hydroxyvitamin D, but for only a few of those 20 were enough data available (i.e., from multiple studies) to enable meta-analysis. Among these final few, Johnson said, the researchers identified three that were associated with all-cause mortality: (1) C-reactive protein; (2) white cell count; and (3) NT-proBNP (N-terminal pro brain natriuretic peptide), which is also a good predictor of heart function and failure.

Finally, Johnson reported, researchers have been searching for functional, or "geriatric," markers of healthy aging. As an example, she described a literature review conducted by John Mather's group at Newcastle University, United Kingdom, in response to a request from the Medical Research Council (MRC) (Lara et al., 2015). The group solicited expert feedback and hosted a workshop, and their work was also overseen by the MRC Population Health Sciences Group. Johnson explained that the researchers developed functional biomarkers of healthy aging in five domains: (1) physiological functioning (i.e., cardiovascular function, lung function, glucose metabolism, and musculoskeletal function); (2) endocrine function (i.e., hypothalamic-pituitary-adrenal [HPA] axis, sex hormones, growth hormones); (3) physical capability (i.e., strength, balance, dexterity, locomotion); (4) cognitive function (i.e., memory, processing speed, executive function); and (5) immune function (i.e., inflammatory markers).

In Johnson's opinion, biomarkers of physical capability and cognitive function are particularly important and are the ones aging specialists "really look at." Poor balance, for example, is a risk factor for falls. One of every three older people fall at least once per year, Johnson remarked, and falls are a leading cause of traumatic brain injuries and hip and other bone fractures. She also emphasized the important role of cognition in maintaining independence.

Where Does Nutrition Fit in?

Johnson then posed the question, "Where does nutrition fit in?" She noted that nutrition plays a role in biological pathways of aging and in prevention and treatment of disease, including obesity. Like Madans, she observed that the prevalence of obesity among older adults is increasing. Not only does obesity increase the risk for many chronic diseases, she said, but there is also good evidence to suggest that it is a risk factor for early admission to a nursing home.

Johnson emphasized that nutrition also plays a role in meeting current dietary recommendations. She referred to Madans's remarks on the overall low quality of the diet of older Americans. She believes that current research on protein could result in a change in the recommendations on dietary protein and noted that sodium recommendations will be reevaluated as well and may change.

Johnson reiterated that a large number of older people are food insecure, a condition that in 2008 characterized more than 8 percent of households nationally (Lee et al., 2010) and close to 30 percent of households in some vulnerable subgroups (USDA, 2016). When thinking about nutrition interventions for biomarkers, she asserted, it is important to ensure that people are well nourished and to be mindful of whether they will benefit from the intervention.

Johnson also encouraged greater participation in the national conversation on health economy. For example, she observed, several of the quality care measures for affordable care organizations (e.g., depression, HbA1c, blood pressure, heart failure, cardiovascular disease) are related to healthy aging.

Finally, Johnson emphasized the need to think about where nutrition interventions for biomarkers fit into care transitions (e.g., when someone is discharged from a hospital and sent home but with no meal support), readmissions to hospitals, and rehabilitation facilities. Although older adults want to live independently, she said, "things happen," and many people end up in acute or long-term care. She also called attention to the existence of a social service health system for older adults that encompasses home- and community-based services, including the provision of meals (e.g., Meals on Wheels). She mentioned an ongoing national conversation on how the medical health and social services health systems can work together and suggested that meals are an important link between the two.

DISCUSSION WITH THE AUDIENCE

In the discussion period following the presentations of Madans and Johnson, a wide range of topics were addressed.

Studying Nutrition in Assisted Living Facilities

There was considerable discussion around the challenge of evaluating nutrition in assisted living facilities and the lack of data in this area. This discussion was initiated by Johanna Dwyer, workshop planning committee member, who suggested the need for more information on this subject and asked how assisted living facilities are grouped in national surveys. She mentioned having recently eaten dinner in what she described as a "very fancy assisted living place" in Boston with a group of people who were all older than 80, including a Nobel laureate. At the table, people were having all sorts of problems eating, she said, either because they had Parkinson's disease, because they could not see the plate, or for some other reason. She wanted to know what is going on in terms of nutrition, she said, "in these very expensive facilities."

Madans replied that she saw this as an interesting question from an operational point of view. She noted that assisted living facilities vary in characteristics and usually are not considered institutions, so the people living in them are not part of the institutional population. Her concern, she said, is that when a household survey is being conducted, the interviewer shows up at such a facility and thinks it is a nursing home, and therefore excludes it from the survey. Likewise, when a nursing home survey is being conducted, the interviewer realizes that an assisted living facility is not a nursing home and therefore excludes it from that survey as well. As a result, assisted living facilities can get lost in the survey process. When she first started working in this field, Madans said, there were clear distinctions between homes and nursing homes, whereas now there is a continuum. She mentioned efforts to define aspects of living arrangements and living places so that data samples can be drawn from across this continuum. Another challenge, she added, is that most assisted living facilities are state regulated. Because of inconsistencies across states, the data on these facilities need to be analyzed in terms of services offered. Madans agreed that this is a growing area in which more information is needed. In her opinion, another area that needs to be addressed is care being provided in the home.

Johnson added that housing with community services can be anything from a U.S. Department of Housing and Urban Development (HUD) facility for low-income residents to a private-pay upscale residence. These facilities would vary widely in terms of nutritional services being provided, if at all.

Sharon Donovan, workshop presenter, mentioned a study conducted in Ireland on the gut microbiome among older adults who lived at home and then moved into long-term care. The researchers found that when people moved into long-term care, their microbiota became much less diverse, as well as more similar to those of the other residents in the facility. Additionally, Donovan commented on what has been learned about the importance of exercise among older adults, for example, with respect to cognition.

The Evolution of Nutritional Intervention

David Goldman, Food Forum member, commented on what he described as the "myriad" of biomarkers for healthy aging and how, collectively, they have been well described with respect to their associations with various conditions. He wondered whether this work will evolve to considering when an intervention is appropriate and how to evaluate that intervention. Additionally, he speculated as to whether nutritional intervention is transitioning beyond simply telling people what they should and should not eat. Johnson replied that a considerable amount of data needs to be translated into action (i.e., interventions that help people), and that there is growing recognition that just telling people what they should be eating is not working. She said that based on her experience, older adults are highly motivated, but that as people age they lose some of their ability to do what they want, such as go to the store to shop. She agreed that the field needs to become more action oriented.

Research to Design Better Nutritional Programs for the Aging Population

Dwyer asked Madans her view on the best way for the National Center for Health Statistics to use additional resources, should they become available, to design better nutritional programs for the aging population. Madans replied that no one thing would lead to everyone living longer, healthier lives. Teasing apart the multiple indicators at play at the national level, including among the oldest old, will require larger studies, she observed. Additionally, while cross-sectional studies are, she said, "absolutely key," she believes the field would benefit from more longitudinal studies. She suspects that people are aging healthier today than in the past. Finally, she called for more studies from the provider perspective, which she said has not attracted as much attention from researchers, or as much funding, as the people perspective. So while the National Center for Health Statistics has started to conduct residential care surveys, she noted, they cannot do so very often, and the result is a gap in the knowledge base.

Sugar, Stress, Raw Foods, and Blue Zone Diets: Miscellaneous Comments and Questions

There was some discussion around the role of sugar in healthy aging and whether added and "natural" sugars differ. Specifically, an audience member asked whether anyone is studying the impact of added sugar on telomeres, inflammation, Alzheimer's, diabetes, obesity, and other chronic diseases in older adults. Johnson replied that generally, added sugars do not function differently from natural sugars in terms of any disease outcome, although she was uncertain about inflammation. The broadest thinking, she said, is that overconsumption of any form of sugar will lead to problems. An audience member stated that it is an established fact that sugar, added sugar in particular, plays a significant role in the development of both metabolic and respiratory acidosis, which she claimed is the foundation of all disease. Johnson replied that excess consumption of any form of sugar can have metabolic consequences.

The audience member then added that, in addition to nutrition, chronic stress and cortisol play important roles in healthy aging to the extent that they affect what people eat and how nutritious it is, and commented on the difference between raw food and highly prepared, packaged foods, particularly with respect to the level of acrylamide in prepared foods. Johnson replied that as some people age, they lose their ability to chew and that certain kinds of processing are among the modifications made to keep food safe and accessible for these people.

Vivica Kraak, Food Forum member, asked whether any lessons can be learned from "Blue Zone" diets with respect to indicators of healthy aging, and commented on how the longevity of people who eat such diets reinforces the need for a more holistic view of physical, mental, and nutritional well-being. Johnson agreed that what is being learned about these communities supports the latter point. (Some of what is being learned about Blue Zone aging came up later in the workshop, in Cindy Davis's presentation on the microbiome; see Chapter 4.)

3

The Spectrum of Aging and Health Over the Lifespan

Session 2 was moderated by Catherine Kwik-Uribe, global director of applied scientific research and scientific and regulatory affairs, Mars Symbioscience. In the first presentation, Janet King, senior scientist, Children's Hospital Research Institute, emphasized the strong connection between in utero nutrition and outcomes later in life. She described highlights of the research in this area and speculated on the mechanistic role of DNA methylation in the link between early nutrition and early health. Next, Luigi Ferrucci, scientific director, National Institute on Aging, National Institutes of Health, differentiated between chronological and biological aging. He focused most of his talk on homeostatic dysregulation, specifically dysregulation of inflammation, which he said can have "devastating" effects, including impaired mobility. Finally, Gordon Jensen, senior associate dean for research and professor of medicine and nutrition, University of Vermont Larner College of Medicine, emphasized that obesity is a much stronger predictor of all-cause mortality at younger than at older ages, and spoke about the so-called obesity paradox—that mild obesity in the elderly is paradoxically associated with lower, not higher, mortality risk.

EARLY-LIFE ORIGINS OF METABOLIC DISEASE AND AGING[1]

King emphasized the strong connection between in utero nutrition and outcomes later in life. She began by describing what she termed the "maternal nutrition–offspring metabolic disease cycle," whereby prepregnancy

[1]This section summarizes information presented by Dr. King.

maternal nutrition affects fetal metabolism and growth and secondarily also affects child growth during the preschool years. This segment of the life cycle is, in turn, linked to the early adult years, when chronic oxidative stress and inflammation begin to manifest. Chronic oxidative stress and inflammation in young adults are in turn linked to an increased risk of metabolic disease at older ages.

The Link Between Fetal Undernutrition and Increased Risk of Metabolic Disease Later in Life

The first evidence linking fetal nutrition to later health came from a series of studies on the Dutch famine during World War II, which, King explained, serves as a natural study of severe food deprivation. From December 1944 through April 1945, Amsterdam was embargoed, and the food supply in the city was providing only around 400-800 calories per day per person, with limited amounts of protein (30-40 grams/day). When the city was liberated on May 5, 1945, the food supply immediately increased to about 2000 calories per day. During the famine, King said, pregnant women experienced severe maternal starvation, and they experienced it at different stages of pregnancy. This event therefore enables study of the effects of starvation at specific stages of pregnancy—for example, around the time of conception, during midpregnancy, or in late pregnancy.

King described how epidemiologists Mervyn Susser and Zena Stein spent many years reviewing data on the Dutch famine and found that not only did maternal starvation have an effect later in life but outcomes varied depending on when during fetal development the starvation was induced (Susser and Stein, 1994). Specifically, King reported, they found that starvation during periconception was associated with decreased fertility, but if a woman did conceive, there was an increased risk of neural tube defects and effects on brain function (i.e., increased schizophrenia and antisocial personalities in later years of life). Starvation during the first trimester of pregnancy was associated with increases in preterm births, stillbirths, and first-week deaths, noted King. Starvation during early pregnancy was also associated with increased obesity later in life. Finally, starvation induced during the third trimester was associated with low maternal weight gain, reduced birth weight in both the first and next generations, and increased neonatal mortality (0-3 months). Additionally, King explained, in contrast with what was observed with first-trimester starvation, third-trimester starvation was associated with a decrease in obesity later in life. King remarked that these data from the Dutch famine show strongly that fetal development is highly dependent on nutrition at all stages of reproduction and that changes induced are irreversible.

While Susser and Stein were examining data on the Dutch famine, King continued, epidemiologist David Barker began reviewing data that had been collected in England and Wales in the 1920s and evaluating the effect of fetal or infant nutrition during that time on health outcomes later in life. In the 1920s, King noted, England and Wales were quite thorough in collecting as much data as possible on mothers during pregnancy, and they followed children's growth very carefully as well. Barker and colleagues found that malnutrition in the womb changes the structure and function of the body for life, making the individual vulnerable to heart disease, diabetes, and stroke later in life ("fetal programming"). This work eventually led to formation of the International Society for Developmental Origins of Health and Disease (DOHaD) in 2004. In 2010, DOHaD expanded its scope to include gestational exposure to overnutrition, as well as to stress.

Barker's initial paper, which was published in the *Lancet* (Barker and Osmond, 1986), was an analysis of large birth cohort studies from different regions of England and Wales. King reported that the authors found a strong geographic relationship between mortality rates from ischemic heart disease (IHD) and infant mortality 40 years earlier, such that higher regional infant mortality rates in the 1920s were associated with elevated IHD mortality rates in those same regions in the 1960s. Additionally, she noted, they found that poor, rural areas had higher rates of infant mortality and IHD mortality relative to urban areas. The relationships between infant mortality and other disease mortality rates (e.g., respiratory diseases, cancers) were not as strong, she observed. Barker and Osmond (1986) concluded that poor nutrition in early life increases later susceptibility to the effects of an affluent diet.

A few years later, King reported, Barker extended his studies using data from Helsinki and examined, in addition to nutrition of the fetus, nutrition of the child during the growing years (Barker et al., 2002). He and his colleagues also had access to data on adult disease. They found that disease risk increased with low birth weight combined with a marked increase in childhood body mass index (BMI) from ages 3 to 11 years (Barker et al., 2002)—in other words, King explained, a child born small but growing rapidly during the preschool and early school-age years. Specifically, compared with infants with normal birth weight and childhood growth, infants born small but growing rapidly showed a 57 percent increase in type 2 diabetes later in life; a 25 percent increase in hypertension; and 25 and 63 percent increases in coronary heart disease for men and women, respectively. Thus, King emphasized, rapid growth in early childhood does have an impact on chronic disease later in life.

Since Barker's initial studies, King noted, more than 100 additional studies involving half a million cases have shown consistent associations between low birth weight and metabolic disorders later in life (i.e., type 2 diabetes, hypertension, dyslipidemia, central obesity, insulin resistance, and cardiovascular disease). They have shown inconsistent associations between low birth weight and respiratory, immunity, and psychiatric illnesses and cancer. It appears, King suggested, that brain growth is "protected" at the expense of lung, heart, and kidney.

In summary, King said, the work of Susser, Stein, Barker, and others has shown that undernutrition during fetal development increases risk for metabolic disease later in life and that this increased risk for metabolic disease is exacerbated by overnutrition during early childhood.

The Link Between Maternal Overnutrition and Later Health Outcomes

Evidence also indicates, King continued, that overnutrition in utero combined with overnutrition in childhood increases the risk for metabolic disease later in life. She summarized some of this evidence, based on a review paper published in 2015 (Gaillard, 2015). Among obese mothers, she said, fetal outcomes include increases in stillbirths, neonatal deaths, congenital anomalies, large size for gestational age, neonatal hypoglycemia, and referrals to the intensive care unit. Childhood outcomes among children born to obese mothers include obesity, adverse body composition, increased blood pressure, adverse lipid profile, increased inflammatory markers, and impaired insulin/glucose homeostasis. Adult outcomes include obesity, increased blood pressure, adverse lipid profile, impaired insulin/glucose homeostasis, and premature mortality.

Of interest, according to King, maternal prepregnancy obesity has a stronger association than gestational weight gain with adverse fetal outcomes. She interprets this to mean that efforts should be focused on trying to help obese women achieve a normal weight before they conceive. Additionally, it is now known, according to King, that maternal obesity alters the placental structure and function in a way that leads to an increased disease risk later in life. She noted that the placenta used to be viewed as being highly adaptable to many environmental conditions the mother might be experiencing. But now, she said, it is recognized that obesity can alter placental structure and function in a way that influences fetal development. Additionally, excessive first trimester weight gain is now known to be a key risk factor for a later adverse cardiometabolic profile in the offspring. Taken together, King said, these findings mean, "You need to intervene prior to pregnancy and achieve a normal body weight."

With respect to the relationship between breastfeeding and later health, King remarked that the literature in this area is not strong for several reasons. First, she suggested, it is very difficult to determine breastfeeding exposures accurately. Many women do not breastfeed exclusively, she noted, and the amount of formula provided is not well documented. Moreover, she added, the data that do exist are primarily from higher-income countries. Nonetheless, she reported, some preliminary conclusions have been drawn: that in high-income populations, breastfeeding is associated with reductions in blood pressure and blood cholesterol and a lower risk of obesity and diabetes in adulthood (Robinson and Fall, 2012), and that early exclusive breastfeeding (4-6 weeks) is associated with longer telomeres at 4-5 years of age (Wojcicki et al., 2016).

Mechanisms Linking Early Nutrition to Later Health

Among the variety of mechanisms that King suspects play a role in the link between early nutrition and early health, she focused on DNA methylation, which she suggested may increase disease risk through gene silencing. She cited two ways in which DNA methylation in the fetus could increase in utero. One possible mechanism, she suggested, is the micronutrient intake of the mother, with folate, methionine, B12, choline, B6, and riboflavin all influencing DNA methylation. In addition, she said, data are beginning to accumulate indicating that the mother's microbiota may produce metabolites with DNA methylation potential in the fetus. She added that because a mother's microbiome is related to her diet, these two potential mechanisms are interrelated.

King went on to describe efforts by Andrew Prentice and colleagues, working in The Gambia, to investigate the relationship between maternal nutrition and DNA methylation. In their first study (Cooper et al., 2012), Prentice and colleagues wanted to see whether they could influence DNA methylation in the newborn by providing women with a supplement of micronutrients prior to conception and through the first trimester. To this end, King reported, they randomized Gambian women to multimicronutrient or placebo supplementation from prepregnancy to the end of the first trimester. They found that periconceptional nutrition did indeed influence DNA methylation in the newborn, and that the genes that were methylated differed between boys and girls. King speculated that this finding might explain why women are more susceptible than men to heart disease later in life. Finally, she noted that Prentice and colleagues found that methylation occurred independently of the season of the year. (The Gambia, she explained, has a rainy season, which is called the "hunger season," and a dry season, when food is more plentiful.) In sum, she said, these researchers showed that maternal diet can influence the methylation of genes in the newborn (Cooper et al., 2012).

King explained that Prentice and colleagues conducted two additional studies (Dominguez-Salas et al., 2013, 2014) in which they examined blood biomarkers of methylation in mothers in conjunction with their diet and methylation of genes in infants. It is during the rainy, or "hunger," season, she said, that the intake of methyl-donor micronutrients is expected to be lower. However, what the researchers found was opposite to what they expected. They found that the blood biomarkers of methylation (folate, methionine, riboflavin, and SAM/SAH ratio [a measure of the amount of methylation possible, King explained]) were higher during the rainy season. Additionally, they found that offspring of mothers who conceived during the rainy season had higher levels of leukocytes and hair DNA methylation. Of interest, King noted, they also found that women with slightly higher BMIs had less methylation, indicating perhaps that they were in a better nutritional state. The conclusion to be drawn from these two studies, she asserted, is that poor maternal nutrition at conception enhances gene silencing in newborns.

The big picture that is beginning to emerge, King summarized, is that DNA methylation increases as a result of maternal diet in utero and that this increased silencing, in turn, may lead to inflammation and oxidative stress. She called attention to the large literature on the relationship between DNA methylation and inflammation and oxidative stress, noting that inflammation and oxidative stress may, in turn, be precursors of aging-related metabolic diseases.

Breaking the Cycle

The question for King is whether this increased risk of metabolic disease can be reduced—for example, by adding micronutrients to the diet. She mentioned Bruce Ames's "triage theory," which predicts that micronutrient deficiencies lead to essential nutrients being "triaged" to support critical functions (Ames, 2006). According to the theory, this shift reduces the availability of micronutrients to prevent oxidative stress and inflammation (i.e., because under normal conditions, the essential nutrients being triaged would be preventing oxidative stress and inflammation).

King decided to test Ames's triage theory using zinc. She and her colleagues fed 18 men a low-zinc diet for 2 weeks (6 mg per day) ("depletion") and then 10 mg per day for 4 weeks ("repletion") and measured oxidative stress by examining DNA damage (i.e., using the comet assay, which measures both double and single DNA strand breaks). They found that during depletion, DNA damage increased, while during repletion, DNA damage declined back to baseline. King described this change in zinc level as a short, acute change and remarked that she did not expect to see this kind of shift in DNA damage with such a small change.

BIOMARKERS OF AGING[2]

Ferrucci differentiated between chronological and biological aging. The metrics of aging, he explained, change very quickly early in life as newborns grow into young children. This early rapid phenotypic change over time then stabilizes for a while as individuals live independently and are able to interact with their environments. Then at some later point, which Ferrucci emphasized is very different for different individuals, phenotype change over time begins to accelerate again. This period of accelerated aging, he explained, is when all the compensatory strategies in human physiology that have been selected to maintain the body's stability start failing, and the body is unable to respond to the challenges destabilizing it.

What Is Biological Aging?

Ferrucci asked members of the audience to imagine walking in Piazza del Camp, Siena, Italy, and coming across a man sitting on the ground, leaning back, his legs stretched out in front of him, his arms braced behind him, holding his torso up, and then wondering how old this man is. There are some discrepancies in the man's appearance. Ferrucci described the man as someone who is clearly enjoying his life. It is a spring day. He is looking up to the sky and smiling, with a pleasant expression on his face. He appears to be past middle age. He has lost some musculature. He is dressed like a teenager, in shorts and sneakers, but, Ferrucci said, he is in fact probably wearing the sneakers because of some pain in his feet. So when asked how old the man is, Ferrucci said, you will formulate a number based on all of this information and say, "This person is probably x." He did not ask the workshop audience to estimate the age of the man in the photo, but Ferrucci said that if he did, the range of answers would be wide. The point he wanted to make was that until recently, scientists were not much better than this at estimating someone's biological age, especially in old age.

If the goal is to develop interventions to slow aging, Ferrucci argued, one needs to be able to measure aging. Otherwise, how will it be possible to demonstrate that an intervention has worked? Based on a review of epidemiological studies, he and his colleagues identified four domains of aging: (1) changes in body composition, (2) energy imbalance (production/utilization), (3) homeostatic dysregulation, and (4) aging of the brain (e.g., neurodegeneration, neural dysfunction, loss of plasticity) (Ferrucci and Studenski, 2011). In his opinion, energy is key and is probably the most understudied and most important parameter for understanding aging.

[2]This section summarizes information presented by Dr. Ferrucci.

Aging-Related Inflammation and Implications for Mobility

Ferrucci focused the remainder of his talk on homeostatic dysregulation,[3] specifically dysregulation of inflammation. The development of a mild, proinflammatory state, he said, is a universal characteristic of every aging organism. He noted that aging has been associated with up-regulation of immune function genes not just in humans but in every living organism studied (e.g., frogs, fish, mice, nonhuman primates). "In every living organism," he said, "dysregulation of inflammation is one of the culprits of aging." Although there are hints as to why this is the case, however, the mechanisms are not well understood, he observed.

Importantly, Ferrucci continued, dsyregulation of inflammation has implications for mobility. He described results from a case cohort study he and colleagues conducted showing that interleukin (IL)-6 levels above a certain threshold (2.5 picograms/milliliter) are associated with higher levels of mobility disability 4 years later (Ferrucci et al., 1999) (see Figure 3-1). "I'm not talking about disease," he said. "I'm talking about something that is really devastating. Development of a mobility disability and the inability to move without help is a "tragic, drastic change in the condition of your life."

Ferrucci explained that normally, inflammation is a "good" thing. An inflammatory response, he noted, is how the body responds to viral and other attacks. When "fighting a war," he said, maintenance and repair are not important. It does not matter during inflammation that one's muscles, for example, cannot synthesize proteins or that erythrocytes cannot be produced or that neurogenesis is blocked (Zonis et al., 2015). It is more important, he emphasized, that the body does what it needs to do to fight off the attack. Then when the "war" is over, he continued, those resources can be used to "rebuild." So when inflammation is transient, he said, "it is fine." Otherwise, the accumulation of damage leads to chronic disease.

Obesity is known to be proinflammatory, Ferrucci explained, especially when fat does not deposit in the normal place, that is, subcutaneously. It therefore becomes strongly proinflammatory because of the infiltration of macrophages and also, probably, he said, because of cell senescence (the loss of a cell's power of division and growth) (Zhu et al., 2009). Yet, while obesity is proinflammatory, he reported, evidence from bariatric surgery and liposuction and the disconnect between rapid weight loss and IL-6 levels in the blood following these procedures suggests that "fat cannot be the only thing" (Klein et al., 2004). Following bariatric surgery, he noted, inflammation drops on the second day, much before any substantial reduction in weight, and following liposuction, inflammation actually goes up.

[3]Disruption or impairment in the ability to maintain a stable equilibrium among interdependent elements within body systems or physiological processes.

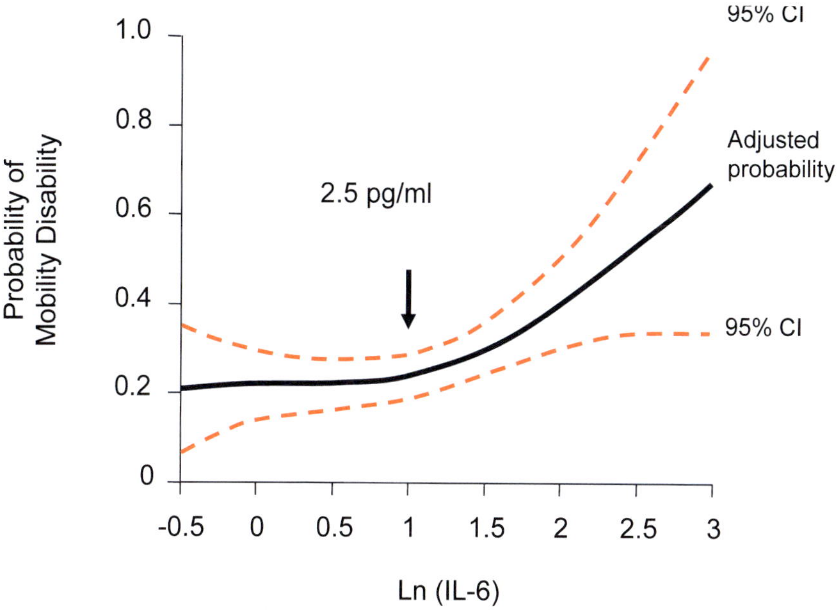

FIGURE 3-1 The relationship between interleukin (IL)-6 serum levels (x-axis) and probability of mobility disability (y-axis).
NOTE: CI = confidence interval.
SOURCES: Presented by L. Ferrucci, September 13, 2016. Reprinted with permission from Wiley: Ferrucci et al., 1999.

Beyond obesity, Ferrucci wondered whether inflammation might be related to the absorption of food. He and colleagues conducted what he called "the fast food study," in which they mimicked a fast food meal (a 1,000-calorie meal with saturated fat instead of polyunsatured fat) and provided study participants with either the fast food–like meal or a healthy meal. During digestion of this meal (within 2 hours of eating), the researchers found a much higher elevation of IL-6 among those who had eaten the saturated fat–filled, fast food–like meal (see Figure 3-2). In other, still unpublished experiments, Ferrucci and colleagues conducted ultracentrifugation of lipids and found that at 2 hours, that is, when IL-6 levels were elevated, there was an increase in oxidized lipoprotein. This finding suggested, he said, that perhaps administering an antioxidant exactly 2 hours after eating a meal high in saturated fat might reduce the negative effect of this meal.

Ferrucci reiterated that during inflammation the ability of muscle to regenerate protein is clearly impaired. He mentioned two experiments in animal models showing that after a meal muscles absorb amino acids for

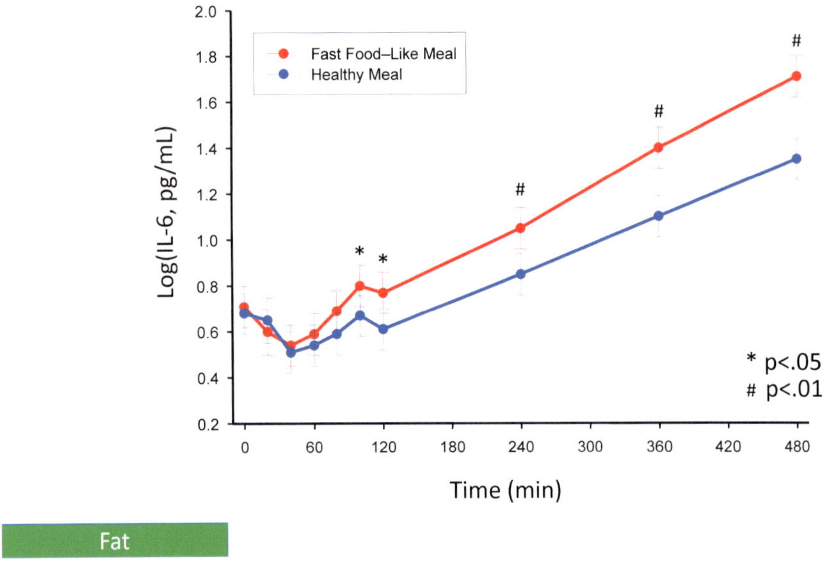

FIGURE 3-2 Change over time in interleukin (IL)-6 according to meal type.
SOURCES: Presented by L. Ferrucci, September 13, 2016. Reprinted with permission.

30-35 minutes, depending on age. In a strongly inflammatory state (IL-6 greater than 3.5 pg/mL), he explained, this postmeal effect disappears. Similarly, in a state of chronic inflammation, the increase in protein synthesis that normally occurs with exercise does not occur. Ferrucci and colleagues found in a longitudinal observational study with humans that in individuals with inflammation, the amount of protein required to maintain stability of muscle mass was much greater relative to the amount required by individuals without inflammation. Moreover, he noted, those with high inflammation, regardless of their protein intake, always showed a decline in muscle mass.

One "quick" strategy for addressing aging-related inflammation, Ferrucci concluded, is to treat periodontal disease, which has been associated with a higher brain amyloid load in older individuals (Kamer et al., 2015). He encouraged examining other "details" of aging, such as the atrophy of fungiform papillae in the tongue that occurs in older individuals (with consequences for insulin secretion), as ways to address not just inflammation but other burdens of aging as well.

OVERWEIGHT AND OBESITY IN OLDER PERSONS: IMPACT ON HEALTH AND MORTALITY OUTCOMES[4]

Jensen recalled that when he first started his aging studies, in the 1990s, he would see patients with severe obesity in the clinic, but that the focus in the field at that time was on frailty and undernutrition. Today, he said, while some frail, tiny individuals will still be encountered in any hospital or chronic care facility, many frail and overweight or obese persons will be encountered as well. During his presentation, he said, he would "wade into an area of tremendous controversy," that is, the so-called obesity paradox, whereby mild obesity in the elderly is paradoxically associated with lower, not higher, mortality risk.

Health and Mortality Outcomes Associated with Obesity

Jensen said, "I sometimes think you are born, you start to have inflammation, and then it progresses the rest of your life." That said, he continued, there are many adverse health outcomes specifically associated with obesity as one ages, including premature disease, functional decline, and shortened duration of life. The earliest studies on obesity and duration of life that did not show a relationship, he noted, were confounded by important covariates, including smoking. It is safe to say, in his opinion, that obesity generally does not confer health benefits. He observed that the classic mortality curve in relation to BMI is J-shaped: mortality increases at either end of the BMI spectrum. Yet while obesity is strongly associated with all-cause mortality, he said, a wealth of data now exist to indicate that it is a much stronger predictor at younger than at older ages. That is, he explained, while obesity in childhood or young adulthood has been clearly associated with decreased life expectancy, the relationship between obesity and mortality in older adults is more complex. In addition, he noted, obesity is associated with a long list of comorbidities, including cardiovascular disease, diabetes, metabolic syndrome, and several malignancies.

The Obesity Paradox

Jensen remarked that the scientific literature on the obesity paradox has been growing for more than a decade and referred workshop participants to what he described as a helpful review by Oreopoulos and colleagues (2009). Although unanswered questions remain about why the obesity paradox exists, he expressed the hope that some of what he would discuss is beginning to provide some clarity. It has been suggested, he said, that some degree of

[4]This section summarizes information presented by Dr. Jensen.

overweight may provide a metabolic reserve for surviving illness and injury, and he believes "there may be something to that."

A landmark paper in the field was a systematic review and meta-analysis of all-cause mortality among different BMI categories (Flegal et al., 2013). This was a large analysis, Jensen said, covering nearly 3 million people and 270,000 deaths. The key finding, he reported, was that, compared with desirable BMI (defined as 18.5-24.9), while class II obesity and class III obesity (severe obesity) were associated with significantly greater all-cause mortality, class I obesity was not associated with higher mortality, and overweight was associated with significantly lower mortality. Among individuals aged 65 and older, the hazard ratios for all-cause mortality were 0.90 for those with a BMI of 25-30, 0.87 for those with a BMI of 30-35, and 1.20 for those with a BMI of 35 or greater. The Flegal et al. (2013) paper, Jensen said, rather than settling the paradox, started a "raging controversy," with a key issue for discussion being how to interpret its findings for health professionals and for the public (Hughes, 2013). Jensen also mentioned another review by Childers and Allison (2010), who showed that the lowest mortality rate in the classic J-shaped mortality curve in relation to BMI generally shifts toward a higher BMI for older persons.

Sarcopenic Obesity and the Obesity Paradox

Evidence from studies on sarcopenic obesity (obesity accompanied by reduced lean body mass), Jensen continued, suggest that the obesity paradox may be explained in part by body composition and that overweight in older adults is protective only in those with high muscle mass (see the discussion of sarcopenia in Chapter 4). One of these studies was Murphy et al. (2014), a modest-sized cohort study (N = 637) of individuals aged 66-96 with diabetes. Jensen reported that the thigh muscle mass of participants was assessed by computed tomography scan. The interesting finding from this study, he said, was that the highest mortality was among those with low muscle mass who were either normal weight or overweight, and that normal-weight participants had a greater mortality risk than overweight individuals, a paradox explained partly by muscle mass.

In another study of sarcopenic obesity, Jensen continued, Bea and colleagues (2015) examined the risk of mortality in relation to BMI and body composition among a large sample (N = 10,525) of women who underwent DEXA (dual-energy X-ray absorptiometry) scans and were followed for 13.6 years. They found that, overall, high BMI (greater than or equal to 35) was associated with increased mortality, while total body fat and lean body mass were not. However, Jensen reported, among women aged 50-59, those with greater total body fat had increased mortality, while those with greater lean body mass had decreased mortality. These findings were reversed for women aged 70-79. These results reflect what Jensen described as a "very complex scenario," with body composition, age, and sex, as well as the population being studied, all being potential factors.

BMI, Metabolic Health Status, and All-Cause Mortality Among Older Adults

Jensen's own research group recently conducted two studies on the relationship between BMI and all-cause mortality, both released just prior to the workshop. Both studies, he explained, involved subsamples of the cohort of rural, older Pennsylvanians with a mean age of 74 at baseline that he and his research team have been following for more than 20 years. What remains of the cohort, he said, is about 2,500 surviving people all well over the age of 80.

In the first study, Cheng and colleagues (2016a) examined BMI and all-cause mortality among more than 4,500 members of this cohort with a mean BMI of 25.9 at baseline. Jensen explained that they followed this subset for almost 11 years. They analyzed three models: one that adjusted for age and sex; a second that adjusted for both of those plus smoking status and alcohol use; and a third that adjusted for all of the above plus blood glucose, diabetic medication, triglycerides, high-density lipoprotein cholesterol, low-density lipoprotein cholesterol, cholesterol medication, diastolic blood pressure, hypertension medication, and disease burden. According to Jensen, the multiple models represented an attempt to control systematically for as many confounding variables as possible. The researchers found that, compared with the reference BMI (18.5-24.9), all-cause mortality was greatest among individuals with BMIs below 18.5, which Jensen suggested may be explained by some of these individuals having underlying disease. In contrast, he noted, all-cause mortality among individuals with BMIs of 25-29.9 and 30-34.9 was lower than that among the reference BMI group, for all three models. At the higher end of the BMI spectrum, he added, the hazard ratios for all-cause mortality increased again. In sum, he said, individuals who were underweight had a significantly greater risk of all-cause mortality, while those with overweight or mild obesity had a significantly lower risk. Thus, he explained, consistent with results of other studies, these researchers found a U-shaped relationship between BMI and all-cause mortality, with the lowest mortality risk seen among those with a BMI of 28-30 (see Figure 3-3).

In the second study, Jensen continued, Cheng and colleagues (2016b) used the same data set to take the analysis one step further and examine metabolic health status (using the Adult Treatment Panel III criteria, with metabolic health being defined as having fewer than two risk factors) and its relationship to all-cause mortality and BMI. Covariates

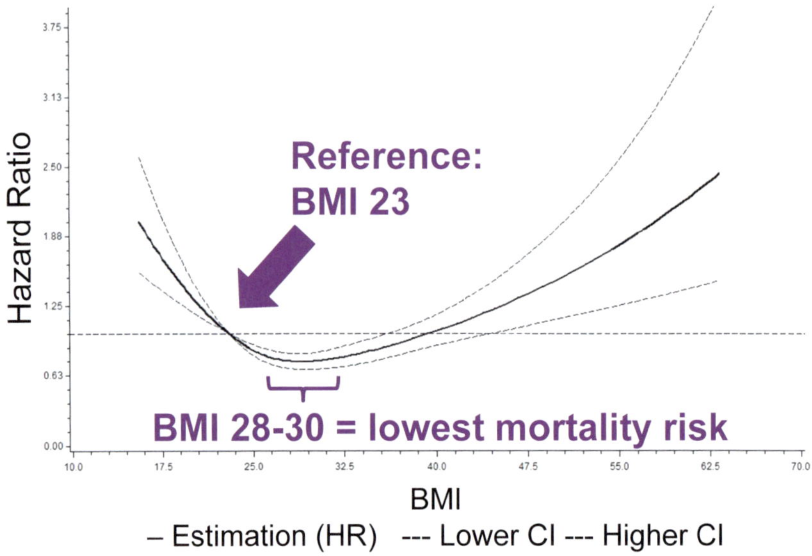

FIGURE 3-3 Mortality risk (i.e., hazard ratio relative to a body mass index [BMI] of 23) as a function of BMI.
NOTE: CI = confidence interval; HR = hazard ratio.
SOURCES: G. Jensen, September 16, 2016. Reprinted with permission from Wiley: Cheng et al., 2016a (modified).

addressed in the analysis, he explained, included age, sex, smoking, alcohol, metabolic laboratory test results, medications, and disease burden. Jensen did not have time to present each analysis, but listed the multiple sensitivity analyses conducted in an attempt to bring a high level of rigor to the analysis, which included analysis of a fully adjusted model with never-smokers with no disease burden; metabolically unhealthy individuals, including all individuals meeting any diabetes criterion; metabolically healthy individuals, including only those with no metabolic risk factors; never-smokers, excluding individuals who died during the first 5 years of follow-up; all individuals, excluding those who became metabolically unhealthy during follow-up; and all individuals, excluding those who used cholesterol-lowering, diabetes, and blood pressure medications.

Over the almost 11-year study period, Jensen reported, there were 2,294 deaths among the study participants. The main finding was that metabolically healthy overweight or obesity was not associated with a significantly greater mortality risk. This finding, Jensen said, was unchanged by the exclusions tested in the sensitivity analyses. Additionally, the researchers found that the association between BMI and mortality was more pronounced in individuals with fasting blood glucose levels greater than 100 mg/dL or diabetes diagnoses.

Although metabolically healthy overweight or obesity was not associated with a greater mortality risk, Jensen noted, the proportion of metabolically unhealthy individuals still increased at higher levels of obesity—from about 65 percent among individuals with "desirable" BMIs to 90 percent among those with class II or III obesity. In a comparison of all metabolically healthy and metabolically unhealthy individuals (N = 4,551), the shift toward an increased risk for being metabolically unhealthy across all BMI categories is "dramatic," Jensen said. The same shift occurs, he observed, in a comparison of only metabolically healthy and metabolically unhealthy never-smokers with no identified chronic disease burden (N = 1,046 remaining for analysis), and again in a comparison of never-smokers excluding individuals that died during the first 5 years of follow-up (N = 2,367 remaining for analysis).

According to Jensen, the results of this second study suggest that there is a subset of what he described as "pretty robust healthy overweight and mildly obese older people." The obesity paradox in previous studies may be partially explained, he said, by the inclusion of metabolically healthy overweight and mildly obese people who did not have an elevated mortality risk. Of course, he added, there are many older adults who are overweight or mildly obese who are metabolically unhealthy and who do have an increased mortality risk.

In Jensen's opinion, an important hypothesis to test in the future is whether these same metabolically healthy overweight and mildly obese individuals are also to some degree protected from chronic inflammation and sarcopenic obesity. He added that the rigorous sensitivity analyses conducted as part of this study show that methodological issues cannot fully explain the obesity paradox.

Conclusion: Benefits Versus Risks

In closing, Jensen stated that obesity generally does not confer mortality or health benefits. However, he believes the current use of the National Institutes of Health BMI guidelines warrants reevaluation for older persons. He said he is concerned when he sees a frail older person in a chronic care facility who is overweight or mildly obese placed on a restricted diet and encouraged to lose weight. With respect to the protective effect of elevated BMI, he believes that both disease burden and body composition are key factors, and that elevated BMI may have no protective effect in the presence of reduced muscle mass (sarcopenic obesity). Finally, he reiterated the importance of determining how to interpret findings on the obesity paradox for health professionals and the public. He said the message cannot be that people all should go out and eat what they want or that there is no need to engage in exercise.

DISCUSSION WITH THE AUDIENCE

Questions About the Obesity Paradox

Following Jensen's talk, he, King, and Ferrucci participated in an open discussion with the audience. The majority of the discussion revolved around Jensen's presentation on the obesity paradox. Catherine Kwik-Uribe asked whether obesity is more of a spectrum condition and whether Jensen or others have examined the onset of overweight or obesity and its relationship to mortality risk. Jensen replied that answering this question would require a large enough cohort of people who have become overweight or obese later in life, and that at present, there are not enough data available to address the question. He suspects that many of the older adults that he and his group have been following were overweight or obese in middle age or younger. He noted the many changes that occur in postmenopausal women in particular.

Jensen does think that obesity encompasses a spectrum of nutrition concerns. He pointed to the range in nutritional status among overweight and obese persons as an example. He and his research team have documented multiple micronutrient deficiencies in overweight and obese older individuals. It is very possible, he said, to be large, mobility-limited, and homebound and undernourished at the same time.

Simin Meydani, a workshop participant, asked whether Jensen would still recommend that older adults stay within a BMI range of 18.5-24.9, given that it appears that only a small percentage of older people are overweight or obese and metabolically healthy. Jensen replied that it is an important observation that some 30 percent of older adults who are overweight or have class I obesity are metabolically healthy, compared with 10 percent of those with class II or III obesity. He clarified that he was not suggesting that public health guidance regarding BMI be changed; rather, he said, "we might want to rethink how we apply it." Instead of suggesting to some older adults who are overweight and metabolically healthy that they lose weight, he observed, perhaps the focus should be on how best to preserve their quality of life with respect to flexibility, transfer, strength, and function.

Meydani then asked whether the metabolically healthy overweight and obese individuals in Jensen's studies were physically active. Jensen replied that the researchers did examine physical activity levels, but only through a single, self-report question. He agreed that this is an important question to revisit. He mentioned again that in his opinion, an important hypothesis to test in the future is whether metabolically healthy overweight and obese individuals are also to some degree protected from chronic inflammation and reduced lean body mass. Physical activity could be examined in that context, he noted.

Several questions were raised about whether and how obesity affects health outcomes in different populations. The population with end-stage renal disease is very large in the United States, according to Johanna Dwyer, workshop participant, with many people on dialysis. While individuals in this population have chronic inflammation and are not metabolically healthy, she noted, the advantage of overweight is quite substantial for them with respect to mortality as well as morbidity. She wondered whether that population warrants a different standard. Jensen reiterated that many factors influence the relationship between obesity and all-cause mortality. He described the association as "very population-specific." He recognizes that his own cohort studies focus on community-dwelling, older individuals, although many are significant health care consumers. Regarding inflammation in people on dialysis, he wondered whether dialysis itself was proinflammatory in some way. Given that many of these people are in a state of chronic inflammation and are metabolically unhealthy, he said, it would not surprise him to learn that being overweight or obese provides some kind of metabolic reserve to enable people to get through what would otherwise be a deteriorating course. He added that the relationship between overweight and obesity and mortality not only is population-specific but also is likely individual-specific as well.

Ferrucci remarked that in longitudinal studies loss of weight is an extremely strong predictor of mortality. When people begin losing weight without trying, he said, this can be an indication that they could die within a few years. He wondered whether the effect being observed in studies of the obesity paradox might be a biomarker of less severe disease (i.e., that people are not going to die within a few years) rather than an actual protective factor.

Finally, the panelists were asked whether there were any distinctions between the sexes with respect to the obesity paradox. The most glaring sex difference, Jensen replied, is that in populations of older, community-dwelling adults, there are not many obese men. He then referred to the several sex differences he had noted during his presentation. Ferrucci added that there are sex differences in inflammation and in the relationship between inflammation and obesity. Women have much lower inflammation than men, he explained, but also in women, a small change in inflammation has a more powerful effect on outcome than it does in men. In women, visceral obesity is a stronger predictor of inflammation than in men.

Questions About Biomarkers of Aging

Biomarkers of aging were another key focus of the discussion. In response to Kwik-Uribe's asking the panelists whether they thought any specific biomarkers warranted further evaluation, Ferrucci commented on the emergence of robust biomarkers that track chronological age, such as DNA methylation markers. By analyzing the DNA from blood, he said, one can tell the age of a person within 1.5 years, but when these biomarkers are applied to biological age, they do not work. In his opinion, inflammation is the best available marker for biological age, but even so, he believes it is a much better predictor of short-term, not long-term, mortality. He suspects that many biomarkers of aging that have been studied in animals and are now being examined in humans, such as the number of senescence cells in the skin, the ability to repair DNA, and the functioning of mitochondria in the muscle, eventually will not only emerge as predictors of biological aging but also reveal which mechanisms in a specific individual need to be addressed to slow aging.

Finally, when asked to name a function biomarker of aging, Ferrucci replied, "walking speed." He considers walking speed to be the strongest available predictor of mortality, disability, and declining health.

Miscellaneous Comments

In response to King's having mentioned some of the benefits of exclusive breastfeeding, an audience member stressed keeping in mind as well the importance of nutrition and the quality of energy and calories during the third and fourth years of life. She mentioned what she called the "Mountain Dew mouth study," which showed that children in West Virginia who consume large quantities of calories from Mountain Dew grow up to have high incidences of oral cavity cancer, neck cancer, and brain cancer.

This audience member also commented on some of what Ferrucci had discussed about inflammation and obesity. In her opinion, obesity is not the origin of inflammation; rather, the origin of inflammation is the level of oxygen in the blood. Glucose sucks the oxygen from the blood, she said, which causes not just inflammation, but also an accumulation of plaque in the arteries.

4

Changes in Organ Systems Over the Lifespan

Moderated by Regina Tan, director, Office of Food Safety, Food and Nutrition Service, U.S. Department of Agriculture (USDA), and Sharon Ross, program director, Nutrition Science Research Group, Division of Cancer Prevention, National Cancer Institute, National Institutes of Health (NIH), Session 3 examined changes that occur with aging in the cardiovascular system, in the skeletal and muscular systems, in sensory and oral health, and in gastrointestinal health, as well as the role of nutrition in these changes.

First, focusing on the cardiovascular system, Tamara Harris, senior investigator and chief, Interdisciplinary Studies of Aging Section, Laboratory of Epidemiology and Population Sciences, National Institute on Aging, NIH, emphasized that separating cardiovascular disease from aging-related cardiovascular change is difficult, as both can lead to the same end-stage heart disease. She highlighted two age-associated cardiovascular changes in particular—atrial fibrillation and hypertension—both of which are common in old age and have unsettled clinical issues. Penny Kris-Etherton, distinguished professor of nutrition, Department of Nutrition Sciences, The Pennsylvania State University, then described recent trends in several atherosclerosis risk factors, and discussed how these and other risk factors in children relate to cardiovascular disease risk later in life.

Turning to skeletal and muscle systems, Connie Weaver, distinguished professor and head of the Department of Nutrition Science, Purdue University, discussed osteoporosis and other age-related changes in the skeletal system and emphasized the relationship between bone development during puberty and later risk of bone fracture. Roger Fielding, director and senior scientist, Nutrition, Exercise Physiology, and Sarcopenia Laboratory, Jean Mayer USDA Human Nutrition Research Center on Aging, Tufts University, then described the many problems that older adults have with mobility and that are related to age-associated loss in skeletal muscle mass and function (sarcopenia).

With respect to sensory and oral health changes associated with aging, Nancy Rawson, associate director and associate member, Monell Center, emphasized that although sensitivity to odors decreases substantially as one ages, there is considerable variation in this decline among individuals and odors, and she explained that this decline is not due to loss in the ability to detect odors. Athena Papas, distinguished Erling Johansen professor of dental research and head of the Division of Oral Medicine, Tufts University School of Dental Medicine, then discussed the loss of teeth with aging and evidence indicating a link between loss of even only a few teeth and lower nutrient quality of the diet, which in turn is associated with increased risk for adverse health outcomes.

With respect to gastrointestinal health across the lifespan, Cindy Davis, director of grants and extramural activities, Office of Dietary Supplements, NIH, described evidence showing that the human gut microbiome can be modified through diet, and explained that gut bacteria can have both positive and negative health effects. Sharon Donovan, Melissa M. Noel endowed chair in nutrition and health, professor, and interim director, Illinois Transdisciplinary Obesity Prevention Program, University of Illinois at Urbana-Champaign, then discussed how breastmilk, in addition to providing all the nutrients necessary for normal growth and development, contains bioactive components that serve important non-nutritional roles, including stimulating development of the gut microbiota, which play a key role in "educating" the immune system.

Finally, Rafael de Cabo, senior investigator, chief of the Translational Gerontology Branch, and chief of the Experimental Gerontology Section in the Aging, Metabolism, and Nutrition Unit, National Institute on Aging, NIH, described several studies in which scientists have been able to alter both the onset and the progression of aging in laboratory animals by restricting daily total caloric intake. He discussed how efforts to identify the underlying mechanisms have led to the identification of molecular targets that can be activated or deactivated by pharmacological compounds to produce the same effects, but without actual caloric restriction.

SELECTED AGE-ASSOCIATED CHANGES IN THE CARDIOVASCULAR SYSTEM[1]

> The greatest difficulty in studying the effects of aging on cardiovascular structure and function lies in separating the effects of aging itself from those of the inextricably entwined disease processes and life-style changes that accompany aging. —Jerome Fleg, 1986[2]

Harris began by highlighting three key messages: (1) it is difficult to separate cardiovascular aging from disease; (2) the changes in vasculature are greater than the changes in the heart; and (3) aging-related cardiovascular changes are common and costly, and they have unsettled clinical issues.

Harris noted that heart disease still leads cancer as the number one cause of death in the United States, with many other leading causes being connected to vasculature (e.g., stroke, kidney disease). Heart-related morbidity, cost, and comorbidity are also very important in old age, she observed, and many of the most prevalent chronic conditions among Centers for Medicare & Medicaid Services beneficiaries aged 65 and older—including hypertension, ischemic heart disease, hyperlipidemia, heart failure, and chronic kidney disease (Chen, 2016)—are cardiovascular-related. Even if one avoids developing vascular disease until old age, Harris reported, the remaining lifetime risk at age 70 remains high for any coronary heart disease, coronary artery disease in particular, hypertension (for which the remaining lifetime risk is particularly high), heart failure, stroke, atrial fibrillation, and obesity (Lakatta, 2015). But separating cardiovascular disease from aging-related cardiovascular change is difficult, she said, partly because both cardiovascular risk factors (e.g., dyslipidemia, hypertension, diabetes, smoking, obesity) and aging can lead to end-stage heart disease and other diseases related to heart disease (O'Rourke et al., 2010). Aging leads to end-stage heart disease through changes in the aorta, she noted, which in turn lead to aortic stiffening and isolated systolic hypertension.

Culling from the literature, Harris listed several cardiovascular changes that occur with healthy aging. These include modest left ventricular hypertrophy, where the heart muscle thickens by about 30 percent between the ages of 25 and 80; left ventricular stiffening, which leads to slower filling and leaves older persons more reliant on atrial contraction for blood pressure filling; left atrium thickening and dilation, which increases the risk of atrial fibrillation; calcification of the aortic valve; increased epicardial fat, which has recently been shown to be a risk factor for coronary artery disease; and changes related to fibrosis of the myocardium and myocyte hypertrophy that make the heart less responsive to stress (Keller and Howlett,

[1]This section summarizes information presented by Dr. Harris.

[2]Harris shared a portion of this quoted sentence during her presentation.

2016). Additionally, Harris noted, there are age-related declines in maximal exercise heart rate and aerobic exercise capacity (total work or maximal oxygen consumption), but physical activity can change these latter two declines markedly. She did not elaborate, but emphasized the very important role of physical activity. Among the several other changes that occur in cardiorespiratory reserve in healthy, community-dwelling persons during peak cycle exercise between the ages of 20 and 80, she highlighted decreases in peak oxygen consumption, cardiac index, and heart rate.

Among the many mechanisms that contribute to cardiac aging, Harris mentioned mitochondrial reactive oxygen species dysfunction, adverse extracellular matrix remodeling, and impaired calcium homeostasis. She emphasized the multifactorial nature of the underlying mechanism(s) (Chiao and Rabinovitch, 2015). The consequences of cardiac aging, she explained, are that cardiac output falls as people exercise, the ability to increase heart rate in response to stress declines, aortic volume and systolic blood pressure increase (but with no change in resting heart rate), orthostatic changes tend to increase, and falls increase.

Harris stressed that cardiac aging occurs in the context of other age-related problems. For example, slower gait speed has been associated with increased risk of operative mortality following cardiac surgery (Afilalo et al., 2016).

Before focusing in more depth and detail on two aging-related cardiovascular changes in particular—atrial fibrillation and hypertension—Harris cited several other age-related cardiovascular changes that she perceives as important but that she would not be addressing. First is that pulse wave velocity increases with age. Harris explained that in younger people, the aorta dilates with systole, but in older people, because the aorta is stiff, there is no dilatation. As a result, the pumping of blood from the heart ends in the end organs, such as the brain and kidneys, leading to damage over time. Second, Harris remarked that congestive heart failure with preserved ejection is a very important disease of old age (Froman et al., 2013). In middle-aged adults, its prevalence is less than 0.1 percent, but in older adults, its prevalence increases to 6-18 percent. In younger adults, Harris noted, congestive heart failure affects predominantly men, whereas in older age, it affects predominantly women. Also in older adults, she continued, the etiology is primarily hypertensive, and left ventricular systolic function is normal, but left ventricular diastolic function is impaired. Additionally, subjects usually have multiple comorbidities. Third, Harris would not be talking about kidney disease related to vascular changes, but noted its importance in old age. Nor would she be talking about the role of exercise and diet in ameliorating, if not reversing, some of these changes; about atherosclerosis; or about inflammation.

Atrial Fibrillation

Harris defined atrial fibrillation as an irregular heart rhythm caused by a disturbance in the electrical system of the heart so that the atria and ventricles no longer beat in a coordinated way. She noted that while most symptoms of atrial fibrillation are related to how fast the heart is beating, increased risk of stroke is an important complication.

The leading risk factor for atrial fibrillation is increased age, Harris reported, which she said is believed to lead to fibrosis of the electrical conducting system in the heart. Other risk factors for atrial fibrillation include hypertension, diabetes, heart failure, valvular heart disease, and myocardial infarction. Not only does the prevalence of atrial fibrillation increase with aging, with rates of hospitalization for the condition also increasingly markedly with old age, Harris observed, but older people with atrial fibrillation tend to have multiple comorbidities as well (Chen, 2016).

Harris emphasized atrial fibrillation for two reasons: first, because of its medication side effects and interactions and higher rates of hospitalization, and second, and more problematic in her opinion, because of questions around whether people who are at risk for falling or have other risk factors for bleeding should be prescribed anticoagulants. Anticoagulants, she explained, are recommended to protect people with atrial fibrillation, especially those in whom it is chronic, against the risk of stroke. But for older people, especially those who may be at risk for falling or have other risk factors for bleeding, the issue of whether to anticoagulate is what Harris described as a "major clinical quandary that has not yet been solved."

Hypertension

The prevalence of hypertension increases markedly in old age and is even higher than that of atrial fibrillation, Harris continued. An estimated 76-79 percent of people aged 75 and older have hypertension (Buford, 2016). In some studies, Harris noted, the prevalence is even higher. She explained that in young, healthy blood vessels, the lumen (opening) is large, and the media (wall) is thin and responsive. In contrast, in older individuals, the opening is restricted, and the wall has undergone many fibrotic changes (Harvey et al., 2015). Additionally, Harris continued, in older individuals, the endothelium (the inner lining of the blood vessel) may be dysfunctional. Other potential changes include vascular remodeling, increased stiffening, vascular inflammation, and calcification. Harris reiterated the multifactorial etiology of hypertension, noting that in addition to aging, other prohypertensive factors arise as a result of lifestyle choices or other conditions.

One of the challenges of high blood pressure in older adults, Harris continued, is that it is primarily systolic blood pressure that is elevated, whereas diastolic blood pressure is usually normal or low. This makes high blood pressure difficult to control because lowering one lowers the other as well. This is in contrast to hypertension in middle age, she observed, which usually involves both systolic and diastolic blood pressure (Smulyan et al., 2016). Also in old age, Harris noted, hypertension affects multiple organ systems. As an example of the many studies on the relationship between hypertension and cognitive change, she cited Buford (2016), who found that people with hypertension showed much greater changes in cognitive functioning 20 years later (as measured by a variety of cognitive tests) relative to people with prehypertension. The author also found that uncontrolled hypertension was associated with greater incidence of physical disability risk.

Harris asked the workshop audience to think back to 1979, when the case for treatment of hypertension in adults under 65 was considered to be "firmly established," in contrast to the "less firmly based" case for treatment in adults over 65 (Isaacs, 1979). The evidence for treating older adults was considered "conflicting and insufficient," she noted (quoted phrases are from Isaacs [1979]). She further quoted from Isaacs (1979, p. 115):

> The prescribing of potent antihypertensive drugs to every elderly person with a high blood pressure will benefit a few, will harm many, and will be wholly irrelevant to the medical needs of most, especially of those in whom the high pressure is an incidental finding and is not the cause of the symptoms for which the patient has sought medical help. We still do not know in which elderly patients hypertension is a disease and in which it is, like old age itself, an achievement. Doctors are advised to curtail antihypertensive therapy in the elderly until much more is known about its effects.

Because so many people who survived to old age had high blood pressure, Harris explained, it was believed that the condition was somehow linked to survivorship and that the brain needed it to function properly. She pointed out that these beliefs existed before any of the many major clinical trials conducted since then had begun (Benetos et al., 2015).

The current recommendation for older adults, Harris said, is to reduce systolic blood pressure to below 150 mm Hg. However, she noted, this recommendation was issued before findings from the Systolic Blood Pressure Intervention Trial (SPRINT) were published and before a recent meta-analysis showed that reducing blood pressure below current recommended levels further decreases the risk of heart disease, and that there is no threshold below which lowering blood pressure does not provide this benefit (Ettehad et al., 2016). Ettehad and colleagues (2016) also found consistency among studies in the effect of treatment, Harris reported, and concluded that drugs specific to outcomes worked, that is, that there is an ability to tailor treatments even within the general guidelines.

SPRINT was an important trial, in Harris's opinion, because it recruited enough individuals over age 75 that the researchers were able to stratify participants by age (i.e., examine all participants versus participants aged 75 and over). In addition to cardiovascular outcomes, moreover, the researchers examined gait speed and frailty status, she noted. The trial was stopped early, she said, because it was so successful. For example, there were approximately 25 percent fewer cardiovascular disease primary outcome events among individuals receiving intensive treatment compared with those receiving standard treatment. The intensive treatment was more effective than the standard treatment regardless of frailty at baseline, Harris noted.

However, Harris said, "We have passed this way before." She referred to a 2008 article in the *New England Journal of Medicine* as an example of a trial showing that treatment of blood pressure in older individuals can be successful (Beckett et al., 2008). It is not clear what the future will hold in terms of recommendations for older adults, she concluded.

THE ROLE OF NUTRITION IN CARDIOVASCULAR HEALTH AND DISEASE IN AGING[3]

Cardiovascular disease is the leading cause of death in the United States for both men and women, Kris-Etherton began, accounting for about 800,000 deaths yearly (Mozaffarian et al., 2016). She described atherosclerosis as a chronic, progressive condition that starts at birth and begins to manifest in the fourth decade of life (Pepine, 1998); 85-86 percent of adults aged 80 and 36-40 percent of those aged 40-59 have the condition. Some of the risk factors for cardiovascular disease are modifiable, she explained, including many nutrition-related factors, such as dyslipidemia, hypertension, diabetes, obesity, and thrombogenic factors, while others are nonmodifiable (e.g., sex, family history, age) (Wood et al., 1998). She emphasized the key role of nutrition in modifying the risk of coronary heart disease.

With respect to how these risk factors affect disease, much has been learned from the Framingham Heart Study, Kris-Etherton remarked. This seminal ongoing study, she reported, has demonstrated how changes in high-density lipoprotein (HDL) cholesterol, total cholesterol, systolic blood pressure, smoking, and diabetes among individuals aged 50-54 markedly affect the estimated 10-year risk of cardiovascular disease (Mozaffarian et al., 2016).

[3]This section summarizes information presented by Dr. Kris-Etherton.

Major Risk Factors for Cardiovascular Disease in Children and Adults: Trends Over Time

Kris-Etherton went on to describe recent trends in several risk factors for cardiovascular disease based on data from the National Health and Nutrition Examination Survey (NHANES), beginning with total serum cholesterol (Mozaffarian et al., 2016). Among adults aged 20 and older, total serum cholesterol decreased from 1988 to 2012 across all ethnic groups, she reported. By 2012, however, as many as 36-50 percent of adults still had serum total cholesterol levels that exceeded recommended levels. The same trend has been observed among children, Kris-Etherton said, with decreases across all ethnic groups but again with about 10 percent of children aged 6-8 and 9-11, both boys and girls, still having elevated total cholesterol levels.

Also based on NHANES data (Mozaffarian et al., 2016), Kris-Etherton noted, about 80 percent of adults over age 75 have high blood pressure. She characterized this high prevalence as "amazing." She pointed out that even in midlife, as many as 54-55 percent of adults aged 55-64 have high blood pressure. She described high blood pressure as a chronic condition that increases with age in the United States and other Western countries.

Another noteworthy trend, Kris-Etherton continued, reported by Mozaffarian and colleagues (2016), is the slow, steady increase in the prevalence of obesity, again among both adults and children. The latest data, she noted, indicate that 40 percent of women in the United States are now obese. During 2009-2012, 20 percent of children aged 12-19 and as many as 10 percent of children aged 2-5 years were obese, a finding she views as "quite alarming."

The prevalence of diabetes in the U.S. population showed a sharp increase starting around 1997, Kris-Etherton observed, and about 6.8 percent of the population had the disease in 2014. Type 2 diabetes has increased in children and adolescents as well, she noted. In 2001, the prevalence per 1,000 youth aged 10-19 was 0.34, compared with 0.46 in 2009 (Dabelea et al., 2014). This percentage is equivalent to approximately 1 in every 500 youth aged 10-19 having type 2 diabetes, she explained. Data from the SEARCH for Diabetes in Youth study from 2001-2009 show this overall increase in diabetes in subpopulations as well: in both females and males; among those both 10-14 and 15-19; and across non-Hispanic whites, African Americans, and especially Hispanics (Hamman et al., 2014).

Relationship Between Risk Factors for Cardiovascular Disease in Children and Cardiovascular Disease Risk Later in Life

Kris-Etherton described evidence from several studies showing how various risk factors for cardiovascular disease in children relate to cardiovascular risk later in life, beginning with findings from the Bogalusa Heart Study showing a relationship between childhood body mass index (BMI) and adult obesity (Freedman et al., 2007). In that study, she noted, only 5 percent of children aged 12-13 in the 0-49 BMI percentile became obese as adults, compared with 84 percent of those in the 95-98 BMI percentile and all of those in a BMI percentile above 99. Looking at this same relationship in a different way, she reported, Nathan and Moran (2008) showed a strong correlation between BMI at age 13 and at age 22, as well as a strong correlation between BMI at age 13 and insulin resistance.

Kris-Etherton described a study that examined the relative risk of various risk factors for cardiovascular disease in adulthood among participants in four different studies of children aged 3-18 who were overweight or obese in childhood. Juonala and colleagues (2011), she reported, showed that obesity in childhood is related to several high-risk risk factors for cardiovascular disease, including type 2 diabetes, hypertension, high low-density lipoprotein (LDL) cholesterol, low HDL cholesterol, high triglycerides, and increased carotid artery intima-media thickness (IMT). She stressed that increases in these risk factors are largely the result of "obesity in and of itself in childhood."

Results from the Bogalusa Heart Study have similarly shown a relationship between BMI in children at various ages and carotid IMT in adulthood, Kris-Etherton noted, with higher BMI in children being associated with an increase in carotid IMT (Freedman et al., 2004). Data from the Bogalusa study have also shown that elevated childhood lipoprotein levels are correlated with adult serum total and LDL cholesterol (15 years later) (Nicklas et al., 2002), and that both childhood and adult LDL cholesterol levels are predictive of IMT thickness (Li et al., 2003). Kris-Etherton added that data from the Cardiovascular Risk in Young Finns Study show a similar trend, with LDL cholesterol, BMI, systolic blood pressure, and smoking in childhood (aged 12-18) all being associated with IMT in adulthood (21 years later) (Raitakari et al., 2003). Even with no risk factors in adulthood, she noted, these researchers showed that children aged 12-18 with two to four risk factors for cardiovascular disease had a higher IMT 21 years later than those with only one or no risk factors in childhood. Additionally, they found that having two to three risk factors in children aged 3-9 was associated with higher carotid artery IMT than having one or no risk factors in men, but not women, 21 years later. Kris-Etherton underscored the remarkable nature of these 21-year correlations. "Even in young kids," she said, "these coronary risk factors take their toll later in life."

Diet Quality and Cardiovascular Health in Children and Adults

With respect to the role of diet in the development of risk factors for cardiovascular disease, Kris-Etherton emphasized that poor dietary habits are one of three major lifestyle risk factors for cardiovascular disease, the other two being physical inactivity and smoking (Mozaffarian et al., 2008). She suggested that improving these lifestyle habits could significantly decrease morbidity and mortality due to cardiovascular disease. She pointed out that the Global Burden of Disease 2010 study showed that dietary risks are the number one cause of preventable mortality, causing more deaths even than smoking (Murray et al., 2013).

Among children, Kris-Etherton continued, only 0.05 percent of those aged 12-19 have an "ideal" healthy diet score based on NHANES 2011-2012 data (Mozaffarian et al., 2016). Healthy diet score is one of seven metrics used to estimate cardiovascular health, she explained, the others being current smoking, BMI, physical activity, total cholesterol, blood pressure, and fasting plasma glucose. She pointed out that of all these metrics diet is the worst. Over time, she noted, children's diets have improved slightly, from only 0.2 percent of children having an "ideal" diet score in 2003-2004. "But still," she asserted, "we have a long, long, long way to go." The same is true of adults, she observed. Although there has been some improvement over time in the number of adults aged 20 and older with "ideal" diets, from 0.7 percent in 2002-2004 to 1.5 percent in 2011-2012, she questioned whether that progress is good enough and argued that it should be much better.

Kris-Etherton remarked that having at least three or four of the seven cardiovascular health metrics "in check" markedly decreases the risk of cardiovascular disease. Today, she reported, at least 50 percent of children are not meeting at least five of the seven criteria for ideal cardiovascular health (Mozaffarian et al., 2016).

Looking more closely at the diets of children aged 5-11, Kris-Etherton observed that only about 50 percent of these children are meeting targets for sugar-sweetened beverages (450 or fewer kilocalories/week), and fewer than 10 percent are meeting targets for sodium, whole grains, fish, and fruits and vegetables (Ning et al., 2015). She concluded that, given the importance of controlling risk factors for cardiovascular disease in children to lower cardiovascular disease risk later in life, "we have a long way to go." In her opinion, added sugar is one constituent of the diet on which "we can really have an impact." She added that children aged 2-5 are consuming

100 calories of added sugar per day, while adolescent boys are consuming 429 (Vos et al., 2016).

THE CARDIOVASCULAR SYSTEM: DISCUSSION WITH THE AUDIENCE

Following Kris-Etherton's presentation, she and Harris participated in an open discussion with the audience. An audience member remarked that infants and small children are not expected to have the same heart rate or tension in their blood vessels as an older person. It seems natural, she said, that as a person ages, just as the muscles and other tissues stiffen, the tension in the blood vessels would undergo parallel changes. If this natural progression could be controlled for, would the standards for older adults change? Would older adults who are now considered "at risk" no longer be considered as such? Harris responded that although it is usual for people to develop hypertension as they age, it is not normal. To support this point, she noted that there are populations in which people do not develop hypertension as they age. These include people who are, she said, "genetically blessed," but also people who are institutionalized and people in rurally isolated populations. So hypertension is a relatively pathological process, she argued, and it is associated with an increased risk of cardiac outcomes. Kris-Etherton added that the current recommendations for blood pressure in older adults are highly controversial, and her understanding is that because of the SPRINT trial, they are being reviewed (SPRINT Research Group et al., 2015), and some new guidelines may be issued soon. Additionally, Harris noted that the first generation of individuals who have had their blood pressure treated are now entering old age. She said it will be interesting to see what happens to the incidence of cardiovascular disease as this population continues to age.

Janet King, workshop participant, thanked Kris-Etherton for challenging the field to begin addressing chronic disease problems in children. She then asked, given how difficult it is for a child to change many things at the same time, what would be the most important dietary change to target to reduce the risk of cardiovascular disease in children? Kris-Etherton replied, "I think that we could do a lot if we could just get kids to start eating more fruits and vegetables." That in and of itself, in her opinion, would improve diet quality and, by providing potassium, help lower blood pressure.

Johanna Dwyer, workshop participant, asked what dietary recommendation Kris-Etherton would have for medicated hypertensives over age 75. Kris-Etherton replied that she would recommend what the American Heart Association recommends—to control sodium intake. It is clear, she said, that increasing sodium intake increases blood pressure, which in turn increases the risk of heart disease and stroke. In addition to focusing on sodium, she would recommend a diet that is low in saturated fat and meets all current food-based recommendations.

An audience member asked about the continuum from childhood through late adulthood with respect to the impact of the Child and Adult Care Food Program (CACFP) on older adults, given that the program is a common thread across this continuum. The questioner was aware of the impact of the program at the 0- to 5-year-old end of the continuum, but not at the other end. Kris-Etherton replied that all programs receiving federal funding should be obliged to follow the *Dietary Guidelines for Americans* (DGA). In her opinion, there is no harm in following the guidelines, and everyone benefits. Harris added that neither she nor Kris-Etherton had a "good" answer to this question.

The final question was whether the HDL/LDL ratio is also a good indicator of cardiovascular risk. Kris-Etherton responded that current treatment guidelines target LDL ("bad") cholesterol, as well as non-HDL cholesterol (all of the "bad" cholesterol, including very low-density lipoprotein), regardless of the ratio.

SKELETAL SYSTEMS[4]

Weaver began by observing that "bone is the tissue that has been thought of to be important throughout the lifespan longer than the other tissues." Osteoporosis has been considered a pediatric disease for many years, while the notion of cardiovascular and other diseases as pediatric diseases is "just catching up," she said. She explained that people acquire 40-50 percent of their adult bone mass and arrive at "peak bone mass" during the critical years of adolescence (Weaver et al., 2016b) (see Figure 4-1). An estimated 60-80 percent of peak bone mass is determined by genetic programming, with the remainder being influenced by lifestyle choices (e.g., diet, exercise). Weaver noted that sex differences in the formation of bone mass include men growing taller and larger skeletons than women, and that "cheating" the bone of its needed nutrients can lead to suboptimal formation of peak bone mass. Bone mass begins a slight decline following adolescence, she said, and the decline accelerates during menopause among women and more gradually among men.

Peak bone mass is important, Weaver asserted, because of its relationship to the risk of osteoporotic fracture, with a 5-10 percent difference in peak bone mass resulting in a 25-50 percent difference in hip fracture risk later in life (Heaney et al., 2000). She pointed out that 30-50 percent of children experience at least one fracture by the end of the teenage years, so fracture in childhood is important; in adulthood, however, 50 percent of

[4]This section summarizes information presented by Dr. Weaver.

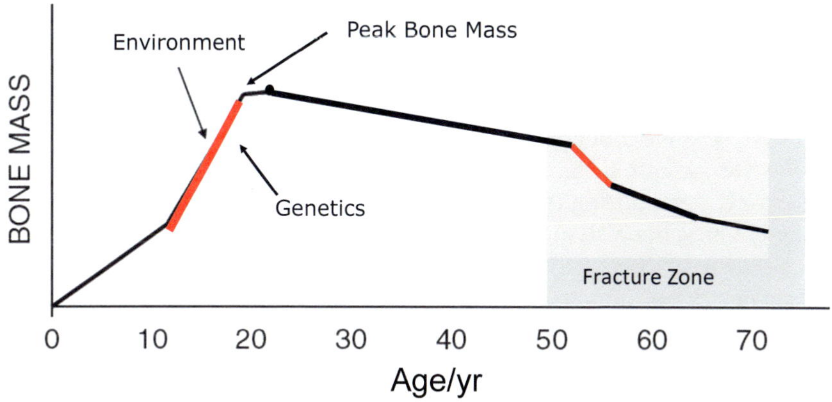

FIGURE 4-1 Bone mass as a function of age.
NOTE: The red lines indicate periods when bone is turning over most rapidly, suggesting life stages for interventions aimed at influencing bone mass acquisition or retention.
SOURCES: C. Weaver, September 13, 2016. Adapted from Heaney et al., 2000, and reprinted with permission of Springer.

women and 20 percent of men over age 50 will experience an osteoporotic fracture. The estimated annual costs for all fractures in the United States exceed $18 billion (Office of the Surgeon General, 2004).

Weaver briefly referred to the common use of bone mineral density (BMD) as an indicator of fracture risk. In adults, she said, the relationship between BMD and fracture risk is linear. She noted that bone mineral content and strength are better measures for monitoring bone health in children.

How Bones Grow

In childhood, Weaver explained, bones grow to become thicker and spongy with greater circumference, acquiring more volume, which contributes to strength. The long bones increase in both length and diameter; their increase in diameter, she said, confers greater strength relative to increases in their mass or density with age. This growth is partially driven, she continued, by sex steroid hormones, which increase prior to the launch of rapid bone growth that occurs around the time of onset of menarche in females. Upon enough estrogen release, epiphyseal closing of the long bones begins, and lengthening ends. According to Weaver, however, the greatest predictor of bone acquisition, based on work conducted in her lab and by other research groups, is insulin-like growth factor-1 (IGF-1). "It is really about growth, or the regulators of growth," she said, with genes related to growth playing a prominent role rather than the calcium homeostatic regulators such as parathyroid hormone or vitamin D. IGF-1 is so dominant at predicting growth acquisition, she observed, that when it is included in a model it plays a central role and minimizes the role of the sex steroid hormones.

Weaver suggested that dietary and exercise interventions may be particularly effective during the periods of rapid bone mass turnover, that is, during puberty, but also during the first 3-5 years of menopause for women (when they may lose up to 15 percent of bone mass) (Hansen et al., 1991). Yet, she noted, no study has compared interventions at these different stages of the life cycle. She called for an analytical examination of this hypothesis, noting that it will probably require an animal model.

Peak Bone Mass Development and Lifestyle Factors

Weaver called attention to a 2016 position paper for the National Osteoporosis Foundation on predictors of peak bone mass, for which she was part of the writing team (Weaver et al., 2016b). Based on a systematic search of the literature since 2000, she and other members of the team identified two predictors of peak bone mass with an "A" grade for the strength of the evidence: calcium and physical activity. The team's literature search amounted to what she characterized as 18 separate systematic reviews. They sought evidence for all macronutrients and micronutrients that might be relevant, as well as physical activity and other predictors. They searched all evidence reported since 2000, which was when the last National Osteoporosis Foundation position paper on peak bone mass had been issued. Weaver explained that the "A" grade for calcium was based on 16 randomized controlled trials (RCTs), 4 prospective studies, and 4 observational studies, while the "A" grade for physical activity was based on 38 RCTs and 19 prospective studies. She said she expects that in the future there will be more studies on physical activity and bone structure (i.e., in addition to studies on physical activity and bone mass), but noted that the tools with which to examine bone structure are relatively new. The writing team found few studies on food patterns in children.

Structural Strength Across the Lifespan

As people age, Weaver continued, their bones thin (i.e., osteoporosis), and the circumference of the bones widens. While the circumference widening helps to make up for the thinning to protect bones from fracturing, she said, it does not do enough to prevent osteoporotic fracture. "The incidence of fracture dwarfs all those other diseases you are talking about," she asserted (see Figure 4-2). She observed that concerns about heart dis-

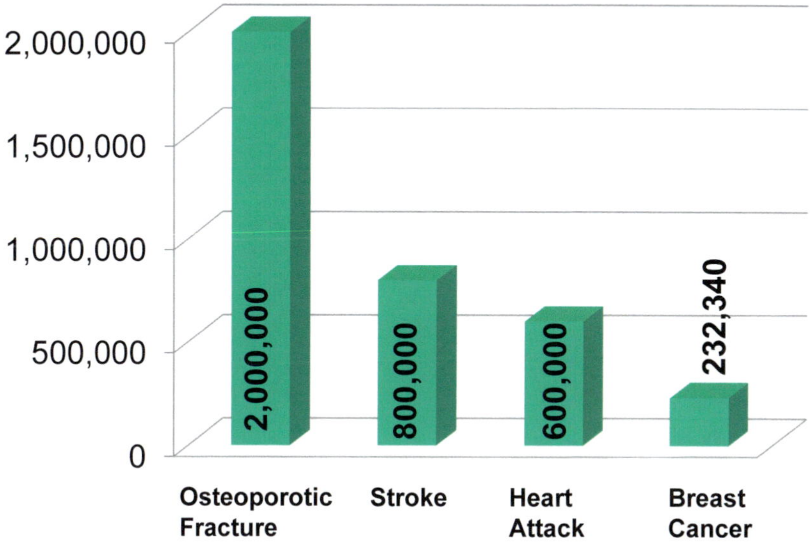

FIGURE 4-2 Annual incidence of common diseases, based on 2013 data.
SOURCES: Presented by C. Weaver, September 13, 2016. Breastcancer.org, 2017; CDC, 2015, 2016; National Osteoporosis Foundation, 2017. Reprinted with permission.

ease, stroke, and other diseases with consequences for mortality are due to their associations with mortality, but a hip fracture has a major impact on quality of life, making a person less sociable, causing a great deal of pain, and dramatically affecting one's lifestyle. In Weaver's opinion, osteoporotic fractures in adults over age 85 warrant more attention.

Weaver defined osteoporosis as the thinning of bones that results from the chronic extraction of calcium and other nutrients needed to sustain homeostatic levels of these nutrients in the blood. The bones thin until the trabeculae are so thin that they snap when force is applied against them. Weaver noted that, according to the most recent statistics (from NHANES 2005-2010) (Wright et al., 2014), an estimated 10.2 million Americans have osteoporosis, and another 43.4 million have low bone mass. She added that the proportion of the U.S. population over age 80 is increasing rapidly and is projected to triple by 2050, which means the overall prevalence of osteoporosis and osteoporotic fractures will likewise increase.

Weaver emphasized the sex differential in osteoporosis, with 80 percent of hip fractures occurring in women and osteoporosis affecting one in three postmenopausal women. She added that the prevalence of osteoporosis is also racially variable: 15.8 percent among white females and 3.9

percent among white males, 7.7 percent among African American females and 1.3 percent among African American males, and 20.4 percent among Mexican American females and 5.9 percent among Mexican American males (Wright et al., 2014). She noted that clinical risk factors for osteoporosis independent of bone mass density include age over 65, low body weight, family history of fracture, and history of postmenopausal fracture (including vertebral fracture).

Current Treatment Options

There is no cure for osteoporosis, Weaver said. All that can be done is to attempt to reduce additional loss and stop the progression of disease. "That's why prevention with diet and exercise is so important," she explained.

Weaver remarked on country-level differences in the 10-year probability of hip fracture in women over age 65 (and with a prior fracture and with bone density test results indicating osteoporosis), reported by Kanis and colleagues (2011). Denmark was at one end of the range (i.e., having the greatest probability) and Turkey at the other. This finding has generated much speculation, Weaver said, regarding chosen lifestyles.

Hormone replacement therapy used to be the mainstay of osteoporosis treatment and prevention for all menopausal women, Weaver noted, until the Women's Health Initiative showed the therapy to be associated with a risk of heart disease, stroke, and breast cancer (Rossouw et al., 2002). She explained that the recommended treatment then became bisphosphonates, which protect against additional bone loss but have some rare side effects that concern physicians and patients (e.g., atypical fractures [Russell et al., 2008] and osteonecrosis of the jaw [Arrain and Masud, 2008]).

In terms of diet and exercise, Weaver continued, calcium (a bone-building nutrient and the major mineral in bone), vitamin D (which helps increase absorption of calcium), and weight-bearing exercise are the most advocated choices for the treatment and prevention of osteoporosis. She observed that, given that 70 percent of calcium in the diet comes from dairy, dairy is an important food group with respect to osteoporosis, and it also is fortified with vitamin D.

Weaver explained that much of the confusion in the literature regarding calcium, dairy, and bone in adulthood stems partly from some of the common challenges related to running RCTs (e.g., unaccounted-for wide range of compliance among study subjects and lack of consideration of baseline status [e.g., a study participant may already have an adequate intake of calcium or vitamin D, in which case providing more will not help]). Additionally, she continued, methods for assessing intake are weak, and life stage, sex, and genetic factors often confound results. In her opinion, results from a Women's Health Initiative RCT of calcium and vitamin D and their relationship to hip fracture "put the thumb on the pulse" of why some researchers report no relationship, while others report significant benefit (Prentice et al., 2013). She explained that among all 68,719 postmenopausal women participating in the study no significant relationship was seen between calcium and vitamin D and hip fracture, nor were there significant relationships between calcium and vitamin D and several other outcomes (myocardial infarction, cardiovascular disease, breast cancer, and death). However, Weaver noted, women in this study were not asked to stop taking their own supplements, and many were taking enough calcium and vitamin D supplements that their mean intakes were at about the recommended levels for these nutrients. Moreover, there was a wide range of compliance among subjects.

Weaver cited a reanalysis of the Women's Health Initiative data by Prentice and colleagues (2013). These researchers found that only women who were at least 80 percent compliant and who were not taking their own calcium and vitamin D supplements at baseline showed a large and significant benefit of the study supplementation over a 5-year period with respect to reducing the incidence of hip fracture. But, Weaver noted, there was still no effect on heart disease. She then cited a meta-analysis of calcium, vitamin D, and hip fracture that included the Prentice et al. (2013) results, which found that calcium plus vitamin D reduces the risk of hip fracture by 30 percent (Weaver et al., 2016a).

In addition to and even stronger than the results of the Weaver et al. (2016a) meta-analysis, in Weaver's opinion, is the fact that the basic structure-function of bone indicates that 36 percent of the mineral composition of bone is calcium. Again, she said, most of this calcium comes from dietary dairy products. Because milk provides not just calcium but all other bone constituents as well (i.e., phosphorous, magnesium), a prudent recommendation, in her opinion, is the daily 3 cups of low-fat dairy product or equivalent (e.g., from a fortified food or supplement) recommended in the DGA. Other "bone-healthy" foods, according to Weaver, include fruits, vegetables, and whole grains.

MUSCULAR SYSTEMS[5]

Fielding remarked on the fact that there are more people on the planet over age 65 than ever before in human history. This is an "astounding" thing to think about, he said. He encouraged greater consideration of the health and behavioral needs of older adults, implicit in which is understanding the role of nutrition. Additionally, he noted, the fastest-growing segment

[5]This section summarizes information presented by Dr. Fielding.

of the older population is those over age 85. "So not only are we getting older," he said, "but we are living to older and older ages." He called for a greater understanding of the nutritional and other health care needs of this oldest old population in particular.

"One of the important things that I am going to try to impress on you is that skeletal muscles actually really matter," Fielding said. He noted that skeletal muscle, which makes up 45 to 50 percent of total body mass, tends to be an understudied tissue in many respects. He explained that many of the problems older adults have climbing stairs, getting out of chairs, and otherwise moving around are related to skeletal muscle, which plays a fundamental role in locomotion, oxygen consumption, whole-body energy metabolism, and substrate turnover and storage. Additionally, there is what he described as "exciting, emerging" evidence that skeletal muscle is a secretory organ, secreting proteins termed "myokines." He described "robust skeletal muscle" as a central factor in whole-body health and as being essential for maintaining energy homeostasis.

Motor proteins and motor functions are ubiquitous across all species, as is the association between mobility and lifespan, Fielding continued (Dickinson et al., 2000). In drosophila (fruit flies), for example, Miller and colleagues (2008) showed that flying capacity declines with aging and that the loss of flying capacity is associated with mortality. This is true in humans as well, Fielding said, with walking speed or the ability to walk one-quarter of a mile being closely related to mortality.

Fielding continued by noting mobility declines in aging (e.g., reduced walking speed, inability or difficulty in walking one-quarter of a mile) are associated not only with increased mortality but also with increased health care costs. Using Medicare beneficiary data, Hardy and colleagues (2011) showed that as self-reported ability to walk one-quarter mile declines (from "no difficulty" to "difficulty" to "unable"), both health care costs and rates of hospitalization increase. Fielding said he suspects that these trends would hold up in many other parts of the world as well.

Sarcopenia

Fielding believes that many mobility changes associated with aging are related to changes in skeletal muscle known as sarcopenia, which he defined as age-associated loss in muscle mass and function (see also the discussion of sarcopenia in the summary of Gordon Jensen's presentation in Chapter 3). He showed digitized images of cross-sectional computed tomography scans of the midthighs of a 70-year-old and an 85-year-old female, both with normal BMIs. The older female has much less total muscle, the majority of which is low-density muscle (i.e., more intramyocellular fat than normal-density muscle), and more intermuscular fat (see Figure 4-3).

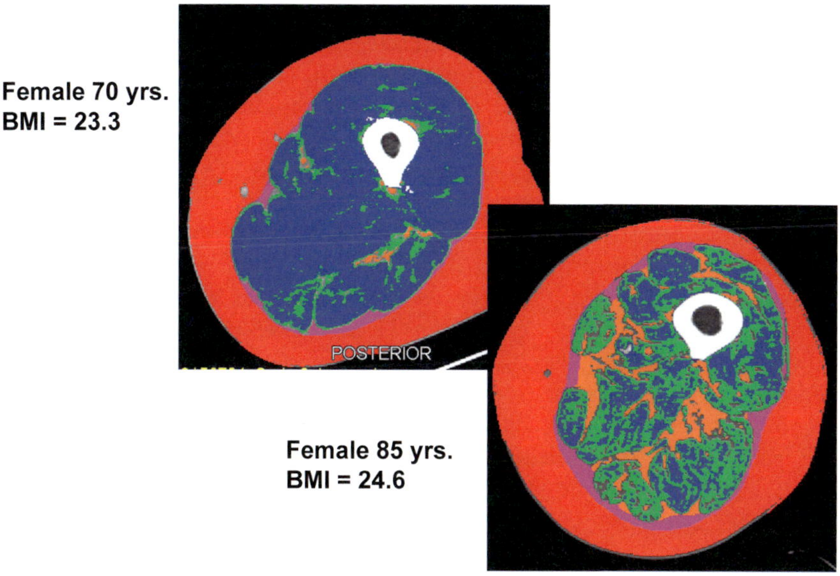

FIGURE 4-3 Digitized images of the cross-sectional computed tomography scans of the midthighs of a 70-year-old female (left) and an 85-year-old female (right).
NOTES: Red is subcutaneous fat, white is long bone (femur), blue is normal-density muscle, green is low-density muscle, and orange is intermuscular fat. BMI = body mass index.
SOURCE: Presented by R. Fielding, September 13, 2016.

Fielding described the images shown in Figure 4-3 as very characteristic of age-associated loss in muscle mass. Additionally, both images are of community-dwelling, ambulatory adults, not hospitalized or otherwise institutionalized patients.

Fielding explained that muscle size is important because it is related to strength, or maximal force-generating capacity. Data from his lab on about 100 older men and women show that nearly 70 percent of the variance in muscle strength (i.e., maximum force that can be generated by the knee extensor muscles) can be explained by variation in cross-sectional area (i.e., of the thigh). Fielding observed that this close association has implications for locomotion and other functional activities as people age. Over time, however, this relationship between muscle mass and strength becomes more complex. To illustrate, Fielding cited longitudinal data from the Baltimore Longitudinal Study of Aging showing that from about age 30 onward, muscle strength (or force-generating capacity) decreases at about a 2-3 percent annual rate, compared with about a 1-2 percent decline in muscle cross-sectional area (Moore et al., 2014). He noted that other studies have shown this same trend as well—that muscle strength decreases more quickly than muscle area. He also pointed out that there is quite a bit of variability in these data, with some people declining more rapidly than others in both strength and cross-sectional area.

Fielding observed that, despite the high prevalence of sarcopenia among older adults (which varies from 0.5 to 13 percent, depending on the operational definition used) (Dam et al., 2014) and the mobility implications of age-associated loss in muscle mass and function, sarcopenia as a clinical syndrome still has no broadly accepted clinical definition, consensus diagnostic criteria, or treatment guidelines. He remarked that there have been renewed efforts in the past 10-12 years to define sarcopenia as a clinical syndrome, and that consensus panels have been organized primarily in the United States and Europe, but elsewhere as well, to develop diagnostic criteria and treatment guidelines for the condition. In his opinion, the most important development in the area of sarcopenia as a clinical syndrome is the October 2016 establishment of an ICD-10 code[6] for sarcopenia.

Definition of Sarcopenia: From Consensus Definitions to Evidence-Based Criteria

Fielding reported that five consensus definitions of sarcopenia have been published, all of which include an objective measure of muscle or lean mass, and all of which incorporate muscle weakness or reduced functioning. However, he pointed out, all of these definitions are based on expert opinion, and only recently have there been evidence-based attempts to establish criteria for the definition of sarcopenia, largely as part of a Foundation for the National Institutes of Health (FNIH) project conducted and published in 2014 (Studenski et al., 2014). He explained that this project entailed a large, pooled meta-analysis of several cohort studies, mainly in the United States, that examined how sex-based muscle weakness (i.e., reduced grip strength) and appendicular lean body mass (ALM) cut points predicted incident mobility disability (i.e., gait speed of less than 0.8 meters/second). From this analysis, he said, two weakness cut points were developed: for grip strength (GSMAX), <26 kg for men and <16 kg for women; and for grip strength adjusted for BMI ($GSMAX_{BMI}$), <1.0 for men and <0.56 for women. Additionally, two ALM cut points were developed: for ALM adjusted for BMI, <0.789 for men and <0.512 for women; and for absolute ALM, <19.75 kg for men and <15.02 kg for women. Fielding

[6]ICD-10 is the 10th revision of the World Health Organization's *International Statistical Classification of Diseases and Related Health Problems*. An ICD-10 code signifies recognition of a distinctly reportable condition.

reiterated that these are the first evidence-based criteria for sarcopenia that are linked to a hard outcome (i.e., loss of mobility).

In addition to gender differences in the distribution of sarcopenia, Fielding continued, most analyses have found that sarcopenia increases with advancing age, with prevalence being higher among individuals over age 80 than among those over age 60. Prevalence also depends on the population in which sarcopenia is measured, he remarked, including such factors as health status, dietary patterns, and comorbidities.

Importantly, in Fielding's opinion, estimates of prevalence based on multiple criteria for sarcopenia are lower than estimates based on fewer criteria. He called for consensus around a universal, single definition of sarcopenia and noted that in fact, initiatives are under way to resolve these many definitions of sarcopenia into one singular, internationally accepted definition. He suggested that another future goal will be to link these objective cut points with other clinically valid, hard outcomes, such as falls, injurious fractures, and mortality.

Multifactorial Origins of Sarcopenia

As with many syndromes of old age, Fielding continued, multiple factors contribute to sarcopenia. He cited decreased physical activity; changes in neuromuscular activity (i.e., decreased number and increased irregularity of motor unit firing); decreased anabolic hormones (e.g., testosterone, dehydroepiandrosterone (DHEA), growth hormone, IGF-1); increased pro-inflammatory cytokine activity (which he said has been shown to activate muscle atrophy genes); and several factors related to nutrition, including total energy intake (Morley et al., 2001).

Dietary and Physical Activity Interventions

Fielding noted that the dietary interventions that have been studied most frequently include those related to protein nutrition and adequacy, either from food or dietary supplements. Additionally, he observed, there is some emerging interest in the role of vitamin D in the health and function of skeletal muscle. Finally, a small number of studies have examined the potential roles of other micronutrients (i.e., those with anti-inflammatory properties, antioxidants, and selected B vitamins).

Much is known about the role of physical activity and exercise interventions in the health and function of skeletal muscle, Fielding continued. These interventions, he explained, encompass both resistance or strength training exercise, which he characterized as probably the most "pro-muscle building" type of exercise, and aerobic exercise. Observational data indicate, he said, that maintaining aerobic exercise throughout the lifespan appears to protect from or slow the rate of muscle loss. Finally, he noted, some studies have looked at various dietary and physical activity interventions in combination. These, too, he said, have shown some potential benefits in slowing or reversing the rate of muscle loss.

In Fielding's opinion, in addition to being potential targets for therapy, some of these interventions may serve as important modifiers of the pharmacological therapies currently being studied (in trials most of which are in early to late phase II). He remarked on the emerging interest in muscle biology in the pharmaceutical industry and predicted that in the future, while diet and physical activity may be used as preventive therapies, pharmacological interventions may be needed for severe sarcopenia.

Protein metabolism plays a central role in sarcopenia, Fielding explained, because skeletal muscle mass is regulated by the balance of protein synthesis and degradation. He mentioned that some evidence suggests that protein intake is inadequate in some older adults, while other evidence suggests that protein intake is related to change in muscle mass with aging. He described observational evidence from the Dynamics of Health, Aging, and Body Composition (HEALTH ABC) study indicating that even within the normal range of protein intake (0.7-1.1 g/kg/day), lower protein intake is associated with increased loss of ALM (Houston et al., 2008). He acknowledged the controversy around "appropriate" protein intake in older adults, noting that the methods for assessing this are challenging (see also the summary of Mary Ann Johnson's presentation in Chapter 2). Nonetheless, he argued, it appears that maintaining adequate protein intake is one way to minimize the loss of lean muscle mass.

Fielding mentioned that vitamin D is probably important as well, based on a preliminary study that he and colleagues conducted (Ceglia et al., 2013). He explained that this study involved supplementing the diets of postmenopausal women who were insufficient for vitamin D with 2,000 international units per day for 4 months. A significant increase was seen in the cross-sectional area of these women's muscle fibers, particularly the type II fibers, which Fielding described as the fast, glycolytic, high-power, high force–generating fibers that people tend to lose as they age. While this was only a preliminary study, he described it as exciting with respect to its implications for the role of vitamin D in muscle health.

Fielding concluded by summarizing his key points: that sarcopenia is age-related loss in muscle mass and function, that several nutritional factors related to protein intake and specific micronutrients affect its progression, and that nutritional interventions may play a role in its prevention and treatment. An important focus for future research, in his opinion, will be understanding how anti-inflammatory dietary patterns and specific anti-inflammatory nutrients influence muscle in old age.

SKELETAL AND MUSCULAR SYSTEMS: DISCUSSION WITH THE AUDIENCE

Following Fielding's presentation, he and Weaver participated in a brief open discussion with the audience. Athena Papas, workshop participant, commented on the concern about bisphosphonates (which Weaver had mentioned as a recommended treatment for osteoporosis), noting that the concern focuses on intravenous bisphosphonates. Yet she said she has had many patients who have come into her office "petrified" and have stopped their medication because of worries about necrosis of the jaw, and she usually recommends drug holidays for these patients. But when she conducted a follow-up study of people she had treated for bisphosphonate necrosis, the majority had died from breast cancer or another form of cancer. Based on her experience, she asserted, people should not shy away from bisphosphonates because of the risk of necrosis of the jaw. Weaver agreed that the side effects of bisphosphonates are rare, and suggested that patients, dentists, and general physicians are all overreacting. She said there is no evidence on the effectiveness of drug holidays or on when or for how long they should be recommended.

Fielding was asked about the role of calories in maintaining muscle mass, especially relative to the role of protein. He responded that a state of energy deficit (e.g., if someone is in the hospital and not consuming enough calories) can lead to accelerated loss of muscle. But a small study that he and colleagues conducted showed that even when energy balance is maintained, a reduction in protein intake still leads to significant muscle loss. Weaver added that the combination of energy deficit and reduced protein intake affects bone as well.

Johanna Dwyer, workshop participant, expressed concern that dietitians and nutritionists are not paying enough attention to sarcopenia. She was also curious about the role of drugs in treating sarcopenia. Fielding reiterated that most of the drugs being developed to target muscle are in early to late phase II trials. He noted that the main class in development is the selective androgen receptor modulators, which act on the androgen receptor but are specific for skeletal muscle, so they have fewer of the off-target effects of testosterone and typically a lower safety profile. The other class of drugs in development consists of those that target the inhibition or trapping of the myostatin protein, a negative regulator of muscle growth. Blocking myostatin action causes muscle hypertrophy, Fielding explained. These drugs are also being investigated for use in treating other diseases for which muscle loss is a secondary outcome, such as chronic obstructive pulmonary disease and heart failure. In his opinion, it will be important to understand how these medicines interact with nutrients, energy intake, and physical activity. Again, he imagined a future scenario in which treatment decisions begin with lifestyle changes, but when people have such low muscle mass that they cannot walk, for example, pharmaceutical intervention may be appropriate.

Fielding was also asked about a comment he made during his presentation on the need for future research on anti-inflammatories and sarcopenia. He replied that some small studies have showed that omega-3 fatty acids can increase protein synthesis and lean mass accumulation in skeletal muscle in older adults. This is just one example of what is known, he noted. It is also known that a Mediterranean diet can reduce inflammatory burden, he said, but it is not known whether that benefit is enough to have effects on skeletal muscle. Nonetheless, he added, observational studies, many of them Ferrucci's work, have clearly shown that higher levels of inflammation are associated with reduced walking speed and increased mobility disability. "We haven't connected all those dots," he said, "but I think we should try to get there."

Weaver was asked whether there are any longitudinal data showing a relationship between intakes of calcium and vitamin D during adolescence and later fracture risk. Weaver replied that better data on this question come from animal studies, in which diet can be controlled for a longer period of time relative to studies in humans. These data, she said, suggest some ability to catch up later from an earlier deficit, but the catch-up is not complete.

AGE-ASSOCIATED CHANGES IN TASTE AND SMELL FUNCTION[7]

In her presentation on how nutrition and nutritional status influence what and how much and how often people eat, Rawson began by describing how the brain receives both external, sensory inputs ("hedonic value") and internal, metabolic inputs ("nutritional value"), and how this information is filtered through experience, health, and age. Sensory experiences are not absolutes, she explained. The sensory experience of bitter foods, for example, is a very different experience for different people, depending on multiple, interacting factors. Moreover, she explained, people's metabolic state can influence their sensory experience. For example, she said, insulin status influences the turnover of taste cells, and hunger increases sensitivity to food-related odors.

Rawson emphasized that food preference and enjoyment represent a multisensory experience, influenced not only by taste (e.g., sweet, salty, sour) and smell (e.g., fruity, smoky, toasty, floral), but also by a chemically stimulated sense known as chemesthesis (e.g., stinging, burning, tingling), the texture of food (e.g., crispy, juicy, dry), vision, and hearing. She noted,

[7]This section summarizes information presented by Dr. Rawson.

for example, that even a wine expert can be fooled by a change in the color of a wine, such that experts describing a white wine that has been colored red use descriptors typically used to describe a red wine. Similarly, a person's response to an odor such as valeric acid is different if the person is told that the smell is from sweaty socks versus a very expensive cheese.

Although flavor is multisensory, Rawson continued, aroma, or odor, is arguably the most informative component. There are thousands of different flavors, she explained, and without the sense of smell, it is impossible to differentiate between wintergreen and spearmint, for example, or between a mango and a peach. Food becomes "very uninteresting," she said, without smell.

Decline in Variation in Odor Sensitivity with Age

Rawson explained that the flavor of food depends on both orthonasal (from the front of the nose) and retronasal (from the back of the throat and nose) olfaction, with the duration of time in the mouth determining how much of a food's aroma actually reaches the olfactory receptors (which are located in the upper part of the nose). By the age of 60, odor sensitivity decreases by 2.5-3 orders of magnitude, with females experiencing the decline slightly later than males and also having a slightly better odor identification ability. Rawson speculated on whether this sex difference is due to differences in attention or experience or in biology. She emphasized, however, that individuals vary greatly in how quickly odor detection declines, observing that there are people even in their mid-80s whose odor sensitivity is comparable to that of people in their 20s. She noted that both age-related decline in odor sensitivity and gender and individual variability in this decline are supported by a history of consistent evidence.

In addition to these gender and individual differences, Rawson continued, recent data show that loss of odor sensitivity in older adults varies among odors, with sensitivity to odors of high molecular weight declining to a greater degree than sensitivity to odors of low molecular weight (Sinding et al., 2014). She explained that heavy odors tend to be deposited more anteriorly in the nose, whereas lighter odors, which are more volatile, travel farther into the nasal cavity. It may be, she observed, that the olfactory epithelium in the anterior region of the nose is exposed to more irritants, pollutants, and potentially infectious agents traveling up into the nose; indeed, anatomical studies have shown more patchiness and more infiltration of respiratory epithelium in the anterior regions. In other words, Rawson said, the receptors may simply no longer be present in that part of the nose in older adults.

Perceived Decline in Smell Versus Actual Dysfunction in Olfactory Sense Identification

Rawson went on to describe a recent analysis of NHANES 2011-2014 olfactory data on 1,281 participants aged 40 and older. In this study, researchers used both an eight-item, forced-choice odor identification task and self-reports of smell alterations. Rawson explained that the self-report data showed it was between the ages of 60 and 69 when most people really noticed that their sense of smell was beginning to decline (Hoffman et al., 2016). When the researchers actually measured dysfunction, however, the largest deficit was measured in the age groups 70-79 and 80 and older. Among the latter individuals, Rawson reported, nearly 40 percent experienced significant dysfunction in olfactory sense identification. When the researchers examined the type of smell dysfunction by age—specifically, whether individuals were experiencing hyposmia (impaired sense of smell) or anosmia/severe hyposmia (no ability to smell)—they found that both hyposmia and anosmia increased with age. Rawson noted that the prevalence of hyposmia was less than 5 percent in those aged 40-49, but more than 25 percent in those aged 80 and older; likewise very little anosmia was seen in those aged 40-49, whereas the prevalence was nearly 15 percent in those aged 80 and older.

Why Does Odor Sensitivity Decline with Age?

Hoffman and colleagues (2016) went on to identify several factors associated with smell dysfunction. Specifically, subjects with a measured smell dysfunction were more likely to be older, male, Mexican American, with a lower income-to-poverty ratio, in poorer general health, not regular exercisers, and heavy drinkers (four to five drinks per day). Additionally, they were more likely to have had two or more sinus infections and to have had their wisdom teeth or tonsils removed or ear tubes inserted. Of these factors, Rawson said, she found the association between smell dysfunction and lack of regular exercise to be particularly interesting, as well as the association with having had ear tubes inserted.

With regard to the biological underpinnings of olfactory dysfunction, Rawson emphasized the importance of hydration in maintaining the right composition of the olfactory mucus, which plays a key role in protecting and transporting odors across the olfactory epithelium. If the olfactory mucus is not properly hydrated, she explained, odors cannot reach the olfactory receptors. Again, she emphasized individual variation in olfactory receptor expression. Another important feature of the olfactory epithelium, she pointed out, is that it is regenerative and continues to regenerate even in old age. That the olfactory epithelium regenerates in old age is "good news," she said, but she cautioned that it is not able to respond to injury or other traumatic effects as well as it does in younger individuals.

In Rawson's opinion, gaining a better understanding of the early development of the olfactory epithelium could help to identify therapeutic approaches to repair of the olfactory epithelium or ways of preventing olfactory loss. There are ways, she said, to culture human olfactory epithelial cells and study their functional characteristics in vitro. One of the more interesting recent studies on olfactory epithelium regeneration, in her opinion, demonstrated in a mouse model that telomere shortening impaired regeneration from injury, but did not affect recovery of cells under normal homeostatic conditions (Watabe-Rudolph et al., 2011). She identified this as an area for further exploration.

As another example of efforts to understand regeneration of olfactory epithelium, Rawson described some of her own research. Knowing that retinoic acid plays an important role in early development, including promotion of olfactory sensory neuron differentiation (Rawson and LaMantia, 2007), Yee and Rawson (2005) found that administering retinoic acid in a mouse dramatically reduced the time required for an olfactory sensory nerve that had been cut to regenerate.

Rawson described as another potential opportunity for therapeutic improvement in olfaction what she referred to as "olfactory training." The expression "use it or lose it" applied to the brain or muscle, she said, applies as well to olfaction. Among both mouse and human olfactory neurons, she explained, the cells that are activated by odor exposure have longer lifespans. She noted that olfactory training is currently being tested in human subjects who have anosmia as a result of trauma or chronic sinus infections.

In their work on olfactory neuron function, Rawson and her team biopsy olfactory neurons from a part of the nose known as the superior aspect of the middle turbinate. She cited one study in which they collected more than 600 neurons from 440 subjects aged 18-88 and individually tested the reaction of each neuron to odor stimuli (Rawson et al., 2012). In so doing, she said, they found something "quite unexpected": from age 50 onward, sensitivities to two different specific odors declined with age, as expected; however, the opposite occurred when they measured the number of olfactory neurons that responded to any odor stimulation, such that as age increased, a higher percentage of cells responded (see Figure 4-4). Upon closer examination, she and her team found that the olfactory cells still active in older adults are those with more broadly tuned odor sensitivities. Specifically, they found that all olfactory cells from individuals aged 45 and younger responded to only one of two odor mixtures, in contrast to about 10 percent of cells from individuals aged 60 and older that responded to both odor mixtures. Given that olfactory neurons typically express only a single type of odor receptor, Rawson and her team have hypothesized that

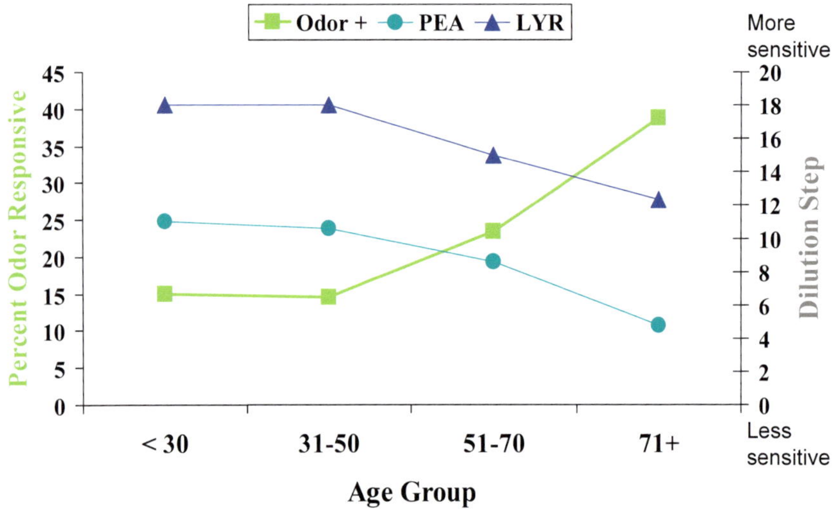

FIGURE 4-4 Percentage of olfactory cells responding to an odor as a function of age group.
NOTE: Odor is any odor; PEA and LYR are specific odors.
SOURCE: Presented by N. Rawson, September 13, 2016. Reprinted with permission.

the olfactory neurons that are more likely to be activated have more broadly tuned odor receptors and that these cells become more predominant as an individual ages. So loss of odor sensitivity with age, she explained, is not a result of olfactory cells not functioning but of a loss of selectivity. Thus, older adults are still able to smell, but they have a more difficult time differentiating among odors.

NUTRITION AND ORAL HEALTH IN AGING[8]

"Previously," Papas began, "old age was 'dentures.' Not anymore." She explained that fewer and fewer older adults have dentures. According to data from the U.S. Centers for Disease Control and Prevention (CDC), she reported, the number of adults who are edentulous (total tooth loss) has declined over the past decade from 31 percent to 25 percent among individuals aged 60 and older and from 9 percent to 5 percent among baby boomers (CDC, 2010). People do not want to give up their teeth, she said, but unfortunately, the teeth they are keeping are unhealthy, with root decay being more common than diabetes, heart disease, mental illness, arthritis,

[8]This section summarizes information presented by Dr. Papas.

and hypertension in adults aged 45-64. In the mouth, Papas explained, it is the root that begins to decay first. The hardest tissue in the mouth is enamel, followed by dentin, then bone, she noted. With regard to dental spending, those aged 65 and older outspend every other age group (Wall et al., 2013), and among members of this older age group with autoimmune disease, dental spending is three times that of their peer-control group because of a lack of saliva.

Loss of Teeth, Periodontal Disease, and Nutrition

Papas referred to two studies conducted in the 1980s. The first, the Nutritional Status Survey (NSS) by the Human Nutrition Center on Aging, was focused on developing dietary recommendations. In the second, the Nutrition and Oral Health Study (NOHS), Papas and colleagues followed volunteers from the NSS, along with additional recruits from 30 inner-city Boston sites, for 3 additional years. This second study, Papas said, was more representative than the NSS of the Boston population, and included more African Americans and people with less education. Across both studies, loss of teeth was associated with decreased consumption of about 20 micronutrients, including calcium and vitamin D. Papas cited another bone density study, in which Krall and colleagues (1994) showed that bone loss was associated with loss of teeth. She explained that as calcium and vitamin D decline, an increase occurs in alveolar bone loss, which in turn has been associated with increased periodontal disease (Inagaki et al., 2001). "Across the board," she said, the nutrient quality of the diet significantly declines with loss of teeth. Without teeth, or even after having lost only a few teeth, she noted, older adults find it difficult to meet recommendations to increase consumption of green vegetables or fiber, for example. Additionally, NSS and NOHS data show that people who wear dentures tend to eat more baked desserts, chips and crackers, and refined carbohydrates. Denture wearers also have lower weights and skinfold-test results and lower levels of plasma albumin, carotenoids, and vitamin B12. In sum, Papas said, "The nutrient quality of the diet significantly goes down as you lose teeth," and this, in turn, increases the risks for stroke, coronary heart disease, and diabetes (Lara et al., 2014). She added that denture wearers may also be at increased risk for cancer, osteoporosis, and other diseases that are already common in elderly populations.

As part of the NOHS, Papas and colleagues examined periodontal disease in addition to loss of teeth and found that people with periodontal disease consumed less fiber. She interpreted this to mean that diet is affected even before tooth loss. She noted that periodontal disease has also been associated with decreased vitamin C intake, and although she has seen only one case of scurvy in her life, she commented on the horrible gum disease with which it is associated.

Papas continued by observing that loss of teeth itself has been associated with increased risks for high blood pressure, high waste circumference, and metabolic syndrome (Zhu and Hollis, 2015). Compared with study participants with full dentition, she reported, the odds of metabolic syndrome were 79 percent higher in edentulous participants.

Papas emphasized that the link between oral disease and nutrition goes both ways. Periodontal disease and loss of teeth affect nutrition, she said, and nutrition affects periodontal disease and loss of teeth.

Medication-Induced Xerostomia (Dry Mouth), Saliva, and Nutrition

According to CDC data, Papas reported, 88 percent of people aged 60 and older are taking medications. In a study of medication-induced xerostomia (dry mouth), she and colleagues compared older adults in inner-city Boston (N = 1,058) taking versus not taking medications and found that the former had fewer teeth and that those taking multiple medications had more root decay. Using the Block food frequency questionnaire, with the addition of the 100 most frequently eaten carbohydrates, they found that, compared with healthy individuals, people who were taking psychiatric medications ate more cakes, cookies, and ice cream (because the sugar made them feel better, Papas explained) and more candies as well (to alleviate medication-induced xerostomia). Psychiatric medications, previous caries, and sugar all were identified as significant predictors of caries incidence. In this same study, Papas and colleagues also found that periodontal disease was highest among adults with diabetes or metabolic syndrome. Among the medicated individuals (N = 980), those who took a multivitamin or supplemented their diet with calcium experienced less severe increases in periodontal disease, and intake of both too little and too much vitamin A was detrimental. Papas said she suspected that high vitamin A intake was detrimental because of its effect on bone density.

Generally, Papas continued, reduced salivary flow results in increased infection (e.g., candidiasis), loss of remineralization (which results in dental caries), and decreased lubrication (which can cause trouble swallowing). She and her research team have been studying Sjögren's disease, an autoimmune disease that leads to the loss of saliva and can cause the salivary glands to swell. It affects women nine times more frequently than men, and up to 4 million American women are living with the disease. Papas explained that with the loss of saliva, what is supposed to be water in the mouth turns into mucus, decay increases, and acid reflux increases to the point where pulp becomes exposed. The Sjögren's population consumes a great deal of sugar, she noted, again because it makes them feel better.

Papas described some of what she and her research team have learned about the oral microbiome in individuals with Sjögren's. Compared with healthy individuals and those with periodontitis, she explained, people with Sjögren's have fewer microbial organisms in their mouths. Individuals with periodontitis have the greatest number of microbial organisms. They have what Papas described as the "red complex," a group of bacteria that have been associated with heart disease. Sjögren's individuals, in contrast, have no red complex bacteria. These individuals get "long in the tooth," Papas said, not because of deep pockets but because of recession and inflammation. She and her team found two potential oral microbiome biomarkers for Sjögren's. One of these, *Veillonella parvula*, she explained, is not a pathogen itself; rather, it augments the actions of accompanying pathogens.

In addition to their studies on the microbiome in individuals with Sjögren's, after finding that some individuals with Sjögren's were omega-3 deficient, Papas and her team tested the effect of an omega-3 fatty acid intervention. They found that this intervention helped with periodontal pockets, dry eyes, and dry mouth.

Loss of Teeth and Survival

Based on NSS data, Papas reported, loss of dentition affects not only morbidity but also mortality. NOHS data show that people who died had fewer teeth than those who did not die. Papas observed that having 23 or more teeth, and having the posterior pairs in particular, appears to make a difference in terms of mortality. Other national studies have verified, she said, that as the number of teeth decreases, so does survival.

SENSORY AND ORAL HEALTH: DISCUSSION WITH THE AUDIENCE

Following Papas's talk, she and Rawson participated in an open discussion with the audience. An audience member remarked on the lack of knowledge about nutrition and oral health in older women. Additionally, she observed that in assisted living facilities people with poor oral health often cover their mouths when they eat or do not even go down to the dining hall because they are in pain or too embarrassed. This relates to both their nutritional well-being and their isolation and depression, she said. She continued by noting that interviews with health workers in nursing homes reveal that they would rather change a bedpan than clean a patient's dentures. In these settings, she said, oral health is not being addressed. Cognitive impairment adds to the challenge, she argued, with individuals becoming combative when approached on the subject. The audience member remarked that some individuals who become combative may be in pain, but the pain is not addressed; instead, they are treated with antipsychotics. She stressed the importance of these issues and the need to raise awareness.

Papas replied that 20 years ago, she and colleagues examined people in 28 nursing homes and found severe dental problems. What bothers her now, she said, is that "nothing has changed." She commented on ongoing work to include oral health in the nursing curriculum so that nurses can examine patients' mouths and address these problems. In the past, she continued, most people living in nursing homes had dentures, whereas today, a growing percentage of people are entering these facilities with teeth. Another problem, she said, is that most of these people are on medications, and that medication-induced dry mouth affects taste and can lead to caries and periodontal disease.

Rawson agreed that taste is a problem for older adults. Many medications can elicit unpleasant tastes or interfere with taste and olfactory sensory pathways. Dentures block taste buds on the roof of the mouth, as well as the release of aromas into the retronasal pathway. Additionally, she observed that oral radiation destroys taste cells and that it can take months for those cells to regenerate. She said she has worked with patients who would rather starve to death than eat food with no taste.

A question was asked about the link between the presence of at least 23 teeth, particularly the posterior pairs, and mortality. Rawson replied that NHANES data show that removal of wisdom teeth is a risk factor for olfactory loss, but the link is an epidemiological one. Papas added that 80 percent of people need to have their wisdom teeth removed and explained that the risk of olfactory loss is related to the sinuses being impacted, and that is rare. It is more likely to happen with sinus surgery, she said, than with removal of wisdom teeth.

Johanna Dwyer, workshop participant, commented on the number of people who have had head and neck cancer and who, after treatment, have no taste and subsist on an oral nutrition supplement. She recalled how past attempts to make frozen foods taste better with packets of seasonings failed and wondered whether any efforts were under way to customize foods for patients with various oral health problems. Rawson replied that a group of chefs is starting an initiative to develop more flavorful diets for hospitals and health care facilities. She stressed the need to think of these foods more holistically, with respect to not only taste but also color, texture, and other characteristics, and opined that it is possible to improve the overall perception and enjoyment of foods.

A final question was raised about whether there were any efforts under way to cover dental care with insurance. Papas replied that attempts were being made to include dental care under the Affordable Care Act, but commented that it is difficult to obtain dental coverage.

NUTRITION AND THE MICROBIOME[9]

Davis described humans as meta-organisms because of their combined human, bacterial, viral, fungal, and archaeal cells. It is unclear how many microbial cells occupy the human body, she noted, but estimates range up to 10 times more microbial than human cells. She defined the "microbiome" as the collective genome of all of these microbial cells, containing about 100 times as many genes as the human genome; the "metagenome" as the combination of microbial and human genes; "metagenomics" as the analysis of the genetic potential of both the microbial and mammalian cells; and "gut microbiota" as the estimated 100 trillion microbes that live specifically in the gastrointestinal (GI) tract.

The functions of the microbiome vary, Davis continued. Microbes provide the ability to harvest nutrients; produce additional energy otherwise inaccessible to the host (e.g., fermentation of dietary fiber into short-chain fatty acids); produce vitamins (e.g., folate, biotin, vitamin K); metabolize carcinogens (e.g., heterocyclic amines produced during cooking); prevent colonization by pathogens; and assist in the development of a mature immune system.

The Microbiome Over the Lifespan

With respect to which microbes inhabit the human intestinal microbiota, Davis pointed out that the initial gut bacterial population depends on the delivery mode, with new strains appearing in childhood and then again during pregnancy. Adults have highly distinct, differentiated microbiota, she noted, but with diversity decreasing in the elderly (Dominguez-Bello et al., 2011; Kostic et al., 2013).

"Can the microbiota be associated with longevity?" Davis asked. She described a recent case-control study conducted on a "Blue Zone" pocket of people living in Italy, where researchers examined the gut microbiota of healthy individuals from several different age categories, including 24 individuals aged 105-109 (Biagi et al., 2016). Although the researchers found that longevity was associated with an increased number of three health-related subdominant microbiota taxa (i.e., *Akkermansia*, *Bifidobacterium*, and *Christensenelliaceae*), Davis cautioned that it is unclear when during the lifetimes of these individuals these taxa appeared. She called for longitudinal studies to better assess the direct association between the microbiota and longevity.

---

[9]This section summarizes information presented by Dr. Davis.

Evidence That Diet Can Influence the Microbiome

Assuming that the gut microbiota affects longevity, Davis continued, the next question might be whether there is a way to modify the diet accordingly to improve health. In fact, she observed, this can be done in several ways, including through the use of probiotics (i.e., foods or dietary supplements that contain live bacteria associated with health); prebiotics (i.e., nondigestible food ingredients, such as inulin and other oligosaccharides, that selectively stimulate the growth of *Lactobacillus* or other gut bacteria); synbiotics (i.e., combinations of prebiotics and probiotics, with the prebiotics serving as an energy source for the probiotics); and dietary components that have been shown to stimulate the growth of certain types of bacteria (e.g., the polyphenols in teas, cocoa, and wine; spices).

Davis cited a study conducted in a mouse model in which it was found that continuous probiotic exposure (for 11 months) increased longevity (Matsumoto et al., 2011). For 11 months, the researchers fed 10-month-old female mice a chow diet supplemented with a probiotic *Bifidobacterium* species, while controls received no supplementation. The increased longevity associated with the *Bifidobacterium* probiotic was due mainly to decreased incidence of tumors and ulcers, Davis explained. There was no difference in weight between the treatment and control groups. Upon molecular analysis, the researchers also found increased production of polyamines and decreased inflammation in the mice that received the probiotic treatment. Davis cautioned, however, that these results should not be interpreted as suggesting that humans be administered probiotics to increase longevity, given what is known about how probiotics colonize the GI tract (in this study, the mice were fed probiotics every day) and the variation that exists in the composition of the human GI microbiome (i.e., because everyone has a different microbiome, it is unclear how different probiotics will impact different individuals).

There is also evidence to suggest that prebiotics may increase longevity as well, Davis continued. She mentioned a review of dietary restriction and the prebiotic high-amylose starch (HAS), which showed that the biological effects of HAS are similar to those of dietary restriction (Keenan et al., 2015). Because of this similarity, it has been hypothesized that HAS may increase longevity in the same way that dietary restriction does.

Davis noted that evidence to suggest that dietary polyphenols can influence the composition of microbiota includes, for example, a study in pigs on the consumption of cocoa-derived flavanols (Jang et al., 2016). Pigs fed the largest amount of flavanols, she explained, had the greatest abundance of *Bifidobacterium* spp. in their feces and *Lactobacillus* in their distal colon. She added that consumption of cocoa powder also decreased tumor necrosis factor (TNF)-alpha and toll-like receptor (TLR)-2, -4, and -9 gene expression in intestinal tissues, producing an anti-inflammatory effect. As another example, she mentioned "very strong evidence" from David et al. (2014) that extreme changes in diet can affect both microbial activity and gene expression in humans. The researchers examined the effects on microbiota composition of a diet composed of either animal or plant products and found not only that the different diets had different effects on both microbial activity and gene expression but also that these effects of diet were stronger than any genetic effect.

That diet relative to host genotype exerts a stronger influence on the microbiota has been shown in other studies as well, according to Davis. In a mouse study, for example, Carmody and colleagues (2015) compared the microbial composition in 5 inbred and more than 200 outbred strains that were fed either a low-fat, high-plant polysaccharide diet or a high-fat, high-sugar diet. A principal component analysis, Davis reported, revealed that mice on the low-fat, high-plant polysaccharide diet had more Bacteroidetes, whereas mice on the high-fat, high-sugar diet had more Firmicutes.

How the Microbiome Influences the Response to Dietary Components

Davis emphasized the two-way relationship between diet and the microbiome, in that the microbiome not only is impacted by diet but also can generate new metabolites from many dietary components (e.g., equol from soy, butyrate from fiber). Many of these bacterial metabolites, in turn, have been associated with health effects. Davis described in more detail two of these dietary component–bacterial metabolite combinations and their health effects.

First, Davis discussed fiber (food component); butyrate (one of the short-chain fatty acids produced by colonic bacteria upon fermentation of dietary fiber); and the relationship among fiber, butyrate, and colon cancer (butyrate decreases the proliferation of cancer cells and increases cancer cell apoptosis). She noted that, based on results from cohort studies, the World Cancer Research Fund International has concluded that every 10 g intake of dietary fiber was associated with a 10 percent reduction in the risk of developing colon cancer; a dose relationship was also found.

With respect to how fiber reduces the risk of colon cancer, Davis observed that fiber can be either soluble or insoluble. Insoluble fiber decreases colonic transfer time, leaving less time for colonic cells to be exposed to carcinogens, she explained, while soluble fiber is fermented by the microbiota into short-chain fatty acids. Of the different short-chain fatty acids produced by colonic bacteria, butyrate is the most widely studied, she noted, adding that it is the preferred energy source of normal colonocytes, and when normal cells are exposed to it, proliferation increases. In contrast, she continued, cancer cells use glucose as the main energy source; they use butyrate in other ways, including as a histone deacetylase inhibitor, which results in decreased proliferation and increased apoptosis (Bultman, 2013).

One of the most interesting examinations of the relationship between dietary fiber and microbial diversity, in Davis's opinion, is a recent animal study showing that a high-fiber diet was associated with high microbial diversity (Sonnenburg et al., 2016). If the mice stayed on the high-fiber diet, she reported, they maintained this diversity over a number of generations. By contrast, she said, animals fed a low-fiber diet showed a reduction in microbial diversity. If they stayed on that diet, microbial diversity decreased even more in subsequent generations; even when switched to a high-fiber diet, subsequent generations were able to recover lost microbial diversity only partially (see Figure 4-5). Davis remarked that these results have important implications because a hallmark of many GI diseases is decreased microbial diversity in the gut. Anything that can be done to promote such diversity, she asserted, is probably going to have beneficial health effects.

The second dietary component–microbial metabolite combination that Davis described in more detail was ellagitannins (i.e., polyphenols with ellagic acid). These include sanguiin-H6, which is in strawberries and raspberries; pedunculagin, which is in walnuts; and vescalagin, which is in oak-aged wine. All of these polyphenols can be hydrolyzed by the gut bacteria into ellagic acid and then metabolized to form urolithins, Davis explained. She emphasized the large individual variation found by Cerdá and colleagues (2005) in the excretion of urolithin after exposure to foods containing these specific polyphenols. She interpreted this variation to be a result of the large individual variation in microbiota composition and

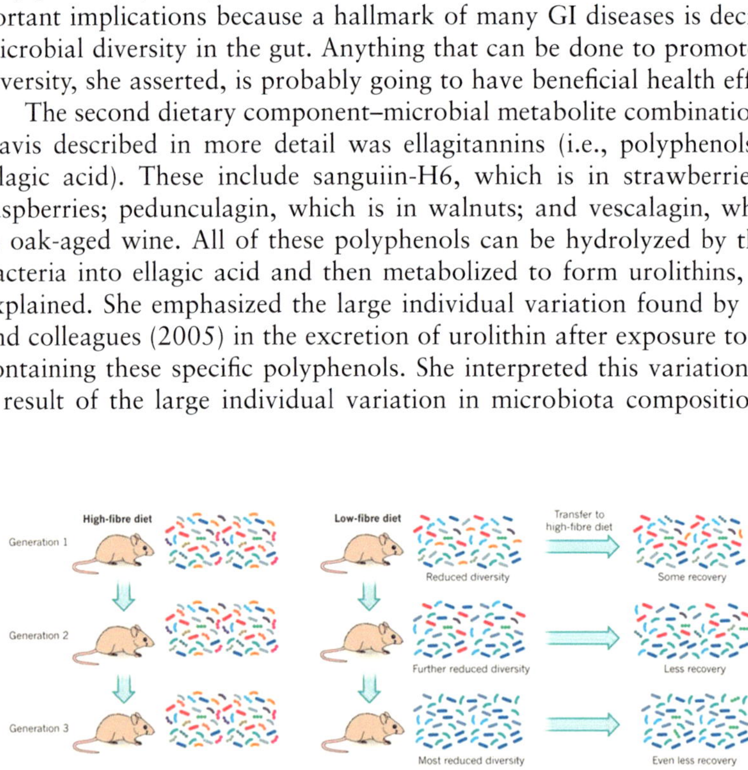

FIGURE 4-5 Change in bacterial diversity in the gut microbiome over time in mice fed a high-fiber diet versus those initially fed a low-fiber diet and then later fed a high-fiber diet.
SOURCES: Presented by C. Davis, September 13, 2016. Reprinted by permission from Macmillan Publishers Ltd.: *Nature* (Martens, E. Microbiome: Fibre for the future. 529:158-159), copyright (2016).

to mean that these same foods have different health effects in different individuals.

In addition to the health benefits of microbial metabolism, Davis emphasized that gut bacteria can produce metabolites that have adverse effects on health. For example, she elaborated, dietary carnitine in meat and dietary phosphatidylcholine in cheese and eggs can be metabolized by gut bacteria into trimethylamine, which is then converted in the liver into trimethylamine N-oxide, a substance associated with heart attack, stroke, and death in a number of epidemiological and animal studies (Brown and Hazen, 2014). Additionally, she noted that mechanistic studies have shown trimethylamine N-oxide to be associated with cholesterol transport.

Importantly, however, other studies have shown that nutrient–nutrient interactions can confer a protective effect, Davis observed. Wu and colleagues (2015), for example, examined the relationship between L-carnitine and trimethylamine N-oxide by feeding four groups of mice different diets for 6 weeks. Davis explained that one diet was chow only, another chow with carnitine, the third chow with carnitine and dietary allicin (a component of garlic), and the fourth chow with allicin. She reported that the researchers found significantly higher levels of trimethylamine N-oxide in animals fed carnitine relative to those fed carnitine plus allicin, suggesting that the consumption of allicin was protective against the production of trimethylamine N-oxide. This type of nutrient–nutrient interaction is not limited to allicin, Davis remarked. She cited the example of resveratrol, which has been shown to have a similar protective effect, and she suggested that this effect may explain the so-called French paradox, whereby red wine in combination with meat consumption protects against cardiovascular disease.

Davis briefly explained how diet may be contributing to human inflammatory diseases. The high-fat/low-fiber "Western" diet can alter the gut microbiota, which in turn can influence the production of short-chain fatty acids and lead to gut inflammation, changes in immune regulation, and altered gut permeability (Richards et al., 2016).

Dietary Interventions to Promote Healthy Aging

Given the dynamic relationships among specific dietary components, the gut microbiota (both numbers and type), and disease risk, the next question for Davis is how this information can be used to develop dietary interventions to promote healthy aging. She described two strategies (Sonnenburg and Bäckhed, 2016). The first, she explained, entails comparing healthy individuals with those having a disease; using a multi-omics-based analysis (i.e., a combination of metagenomics, metatranscriptomics, metaproteomics, and metametabolomics) to generate hypotheses; testing these hypotheses to elucidate the mechanisms; and then conducting clinical trials. The second approach entails providing individuals with dietary interventions, seeing who responds and who does not, trying to identify through computer learning what factors drive the difference between responders and nonresponders, and then formulating and testing mechanistic hypotheses.

This second approach was recently examined in what Davis considers to be the most important paper published on diet and the microbiome. Zeevi and colleagues (2015) collected data on 800 individuals, ran a computer model, and conducted a dietary intervention study, and found that differences in glycemic response to the same foods could be predicted based on information about the gut microbiome. Davis interprets these results to mean that different people respond differently to the same food. She said she envisions a future of personalized nutrition and suggested taking a metagenomic view of the dinner plate, that is, thinking about dinner not in terms of the traditional food groups, but in terms of the microbial metabolites produced from the foods being eaten (Dutton and Turnbaugh, 2012). "When you sit down to dinner tonight," she concluded "realize that you are not just feeding yourself. You are also feeding the millions of microbes in your gastrointestinal tract."

NONINVASIVE METHODS FOR ASSESSING NUTRITIONAL REGULATION OF NEONATAL GUT GENE EXPRESSION AND HOST–MICROBE INTERACTIONS[10]

Donovan remarked that she always likes to start her presentations with a quote from the 2004 Institute of Medicine report *Infant Formula: Evaluating the Safety of New Ingredients*: "Infancy is a uniquely vulnerable period of rapid growth and development and, as such, feeding changes have the potential to impart benefit or harm in the short term, into early childhood, and even later into adulthood" (IOM, 2004, p. 16). While the International Society for Developmental Origins of Health and Disease focuses on prenatal programming, she believes that postnatal programming is very important as well. She envisions that future research will show the importance of the development of the microbiome in early life. Microbes have existed much longer than humans have, she said, so humans evolved within a microbial world. She reiterated what Davis had said about humans having 100 times more microbial genes than human genes in their bodies. Like others in the field, she thinks of humans as having evolved in response to these microbes rather than the opposite, and that many Westernized populations have lost their "founder microbes" through sanitation, Caesarean deliveries, formula feeding, antibiotic use, and other modern practices.

---

[10]This section summarizes information presented by Dr. Donovan.

Bioactive Components in Human Milk

While there is no nutrition facts label for breastmilk, Donovan observed, researchers continue to learn about the components of breastmilk and their functions. She noted that breastmilk is considered the ideal food for infants because it provides all the nutrients necessary for normal growth and development while also reducing the risk of many diseases (American Academy of Pediatrics, 2012). While proper nutrition is critical for normal growth and development, she clarified that pediatric nutrition is not just about providing nutrients. She explained that human milk contains bioactive components (such as human milk oligosaccharides and immune proteins) that serve non-nutritional roles, including stimulating development of the gut microbiota.

Based on what has been learned from epidemiological and clinical studies, Donovan continued, many of the health benefits of these bioactives are related to protection against acute infections in early life (e.g., respiratory tract and GI infections) (American Academy of Pediatrics, 2012). Breastmilk also has the potential to program for longer-term immune-related diseases, she added, such as asthma, atopic dermatitis, and inflammatory bowel disease (American Academy of Pediatrics, 2012). In sum, she asserted, the early microbiota are critically important for educating the immune system—with respect not only to developing tolerance but also to mounting an appropriate immune response in the face of a bacterial or viral challenge.

Donovan continued by observing that the health benefits of breastfeeding appear to be dose-dependent. She gave the example of ear infections, for which the risk is 25 percent lower with any breastfeeding and 77 percent lower with exclusive breastfeeding (American Academy of Pediatrics, 2012). Genetics also plays a role, she noted. With atopic dermatitis, for example, the protective effect of breastmilk is not as great when there is a family history of the disease (American Academy of Pediatrics, 2012).

Breastfeeding also impacts development, Donovan continued, citing known differences in growth between breastfed and formula-fed infants and associations between rapid growth of formula-fed infants in early life and its association with increased risk of obesity later in life. She noted that data exist to suggest improvements in cognitive development with breastfeeding as well, indicating a 6- to 8-point difference in IQ. She suspects that researchers may find other cognitive benefits as well.

Breastfeeding Versus Formula Feeding: The Gut Microbiome, Intestinal Development, and Immune Development

It is important to keep in mind, Donovan opined, that establishment of the microbiome in early life, intestinal development, and immune development are continually interacting. She spoke of the trillions of bacteria in the human gut that are separated from the bloodstream and immune cells by a mucosal barrier one epithelial cell thick. So, she said, there is constant interaction. She reflected that there is no reason to think this interaction does not continue throughout life and that it is probably increasingly important in the elderly. In addition to thinking about the gut microbiome in the elderly, she encouraged more consideration of gut function, given how closely related these processes are.

It used to be thought that babies came out of the womb sterile, Donovan noted, but researchers now know from studies of the meconium that babies swallow an amniotic fluid microbiome that appears to educate the immune system (Rautava et al., 2012). It is when babies actually come out of the womb that they are bombarded with microbes from the environment, she observed, and which microbes take hold depends on host genetics (based on evidence from twin studies), whether the delivery is term or preterm, whether the infant is delivered vaginally or by C-section, and whether antibiotics are administered (Adlerberth and Wold, 2009). Beyond that initial colonization, she continued, whether there are siblings, pets, and smoking in the home, as well as other factors, also can affect which microbes take hold. Finally, she said, nutrition also matters. She explained that breastmilk contains human milk oligosaccharides (HMOs), which are high in concentration and diversity. Additionally, human milk contains microbiota that differ from what is in formula with added probiotics, as well as bacteria on the maternal skin. The effect of formula on the infant microbiome, Donovan noted, depends on whether probiotics or prebiotics have been added to the formula.

A Noninvasive Approach to Studying the Infant Gut Microbiome

Donovan remarked that many studies of the early human gut microbiome are descriptive, with very few having examined potential mechanisms of action. The challenge, she observed, is that no institutional review board or mother is going to allow researchers to biopsy a healthy baby's intestine for research purposes. She went on to describe how she and her colleague Robert Chapkin at Texas A&M University have applied a noninvasive fecal sampling approach developed by Chapkin to investigate what she described as the "black box" of the infant intestine and compare this black box in breastmilk- versus formula-fed infants (Chapkin et al., 2010). Chapkin's method involves collecting mRNA from exfoliated epithelial cells in stool (Davidson et al., 1995); she noted that humans shed about 10^{10} of these cells daily as part of normal gut turnover (Potten et al., 1979). This black box, she explained, includes all of the components of the diet that affect the intestinal microbiota, the gut metagenome (i.e., the combination of microbial and host genes), and bacterial components and metabolites (e.g., short-chain fatty acids) (Hattori and Taylor, 2009). The interactions among all of these factors, she said, influence the balance of health and disease.

Using Chapkin's method, Donovan and her collaborators isolated mRNA in fecal samples from breastfed and formula-fed infants and analyzed intestinal gene expression using microarrays (Chapkin et al., 2010). This was a proof-of-concept study, she explained, so the sample size was small and included only vaginally delivered, term infants (because as noted, C-section delivery and preterm delivery both affect the microbiota). The researchers also limited their subjects to infants of second-parity mothers, a decision made, she said, because they did not want to influence whether a mother fed her infant breastmilk or formula. This study was conducted before prebiotics were added to infant formula, she noted. Stool samples were collected by the mothers at home at 3 months. That mothers could collect the samples is "the beauty" of this technique, Donovan said.

Donovan and her team found no difference between the breastfed (N = 16) and formula-fed (N = 10) infants in age, weight, or length. Additionally, infants in both groups grew similarly in the first 3 months. In both groups, Donovan reported, intake decreased slightly over time while body weight increased, but these changes were not significant.

Donovan went on to explain that upon analysis of intestinal mRNA (the isolated mammalian mRNA were applied to an array of 57,000 genes), her team found about 4,200 genes that showed signals. Of these, her team identified about 1,200 genes with significantly different levels of expression between the breastfed and formula-fed infants. When they queried these 1,200 genes against a list of approximately 430 genes for which prior knowledge suggested differential expression between breastfed and formula-fed infants, 146 genes on this list were differentially expressed and were subjected to further analysis.

Donovan explained that this final list of 146 genes was subjected first to a linear discriminate analysis (to identify which genes discriminate between breastfed and formula-fed infants) and second to a standard gene pathway analysis using Metacore™. As one example of their findings, she observed that the linear discriminate analysis identified endothelial PAS Domain Protein 1 (*EPAS1*) as the best gene classifier, or biomarker, of a breastfed versus formula-fed infant. Several others showed 2- to 5.5-fold differential expression (*EPAS1* showed a 3.3-fold difference). Interestingly, Donovan said, all of the differentially expressed genes were up-regulated in the breastfed infants, a finding consistent with what has been observed in monkeys and pigs.

The network analysis showed, surprisingly in Donovan's opinion, that the strongest gene networks were basic signal transduction pathways. Two of these genes, *WNT* and *NOTCH*, are expressed in the intestinal stem cells and function as fundamental genes in gut development. *WNT* regulates cell proliferation, and *NOTCH* is a differentiation factor. These genes are clearly important in early life, Donovan said. Other networks of expected genes also emerged (e.g., genes involved with inflammation) (Chapkin et al., 2010).

In summary, Donovan said that her team was able to show in this study that the relationship between diet and host gene expression in infants can be assessed using a completely noninvasive technique. They identified some two- and three-gene combinations that could serve as potential biomarkers of breastfeeding versus formula feeding in infants. The differentially expressed genes not only provide insight into potential mechanisms whereby human milk regulates intestinal development, but also represent potential targets for manipulation of the composition of infant formula. While she did not have time to elaborate, Donovan mentioned having used the same approach to show developmental differences in gene expression between preterm and term infants (Knight et al., 2014).

As described in a more recent paper (Wang et al., 2015), Donovan and colleagues also examined the microbiota in the same infants studied by Chapkin and colleagues (2010). This time, they used pyrosequencing to analyze bacterial 16s rRNA. The main finding, Donovan said, was that the breastfed versus formula-fed bacterial sequences were clustered separately, but with much more variability among the breastfed than among the formula-fed infants. When the researchers examined particular groups of microbes, she reported, they found at the phyla level that 50 percent of the bacteria in both groups were Actinobacteria (e.g., *Bifidobacterium* sp.). In contrast, the gut microbiota of adults are dominated by bacteria belonging to the Firmicutes and Bacteroidetes phyla. Interestingly, in Donovan's opinion, she and her team found that breastfed infants had significantly more Bacteroidetes relative to formula-fed infants but significantly fewer Firmicutes. She noted that other work (in Jeffrey Gordon's lab at Washington University) has shown that a higher ratio of Firmicutes to Bacteroidetes is potentially obesogenic, suggesting to her that the observed ratio in this study (i.e., in the formula-fed infants) may be indicative of early-life programming of obesogenic pathways. These researchers identified five distinct signatures based on the percentage of total classified microbes within each of five phyla (Actinobacteria, Firmicutes, Bacteroidetes, Proteobacteria, and Verrucomicrobia) (see Figure 4-6). That all of the formula-fed infants had the same signature (FF in Figure 4-6), while the breastfed infants had one

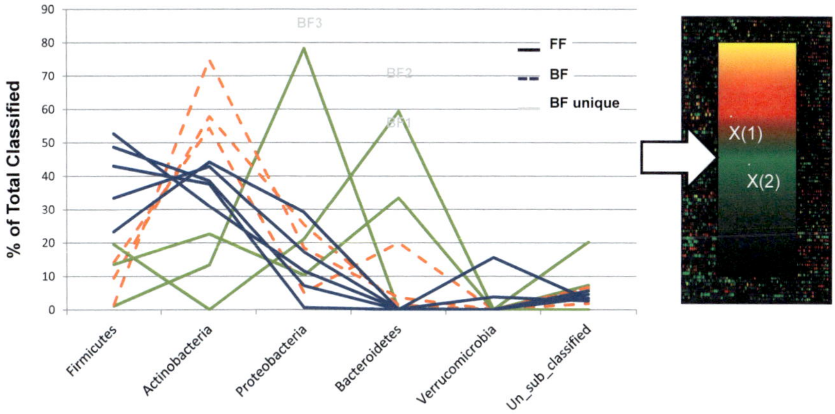

FIGURE 4-6 Percentages of five phyla found in the gut microbiota of breastfed (BF) and formula-fed (FF) infants.
NOTES: Each line represents the microbiota from a single infant. "BF unique" (green lines) indicates phyla "signatures" that are distinctly different from the general trend among BF infants (orange lines).
SOURCE: Presented by S. Donovan, September 13, 2016.

of four distinct signatures (BB, BF1, BF2, or BF3 in Figure 4-6), means, Donovan explained, that although these infants were genetically different, formula feeding was driving their microbial composition, at least at the phylum level, to be very similar.

Based on these differences in microbiota composition and infant exfoliated cell gene expression, Donovan and Chapkin next examined the relationship between host and microbial gene expression (Schwartz et al., 2012). The one category of genes that were differentially expressed in the microbiota of breastfed versus formula-fed infants was "virulence" genes (Schwartz et al., 2012). Donovan and her team found a statistically significant relationship between virulence genes in the microbiota and immunity and defense genes expressed in the infant epithelial cells. According to Donovan, the Schwartz et al. (2012) study documents the first demonstration that virulence genes in the microbiota are actually communicating in some way with and influencing the expression of immunity and defense genes in the infant, with the net effect being down-regulation of inflammatory genes in the gut.

THE GUT AND GUT MICROBIOME: DISCUSSION WITH THE AUDIENCE

Following Donovan's talk, she and Davis participated in an open discussion with the audience. Duffy Mackay, workshop presenter, asked about the significance of the metagenome: Are host mechanics reading microbial genes? Or are host signal molecules regulating microbial genes, or vice versa? Davis responded that the metagenome provides information about the potential interactions between the host and the microbiome. Both influence each other, she said. Donovan added that researchers are also beginning to examine the metatranscriptome, that is, the microbial mRNA, which she said is a "little trickier." She explained that mRNA is not as stable as DNA; however, it provides a closer picture of how the bacteria are actually functioning. She reiterated that it is known that diet can change the metagenome and predicted that over time, it will become clear that the products of microbial metabolism are critically important in signaling to the host. Davis added that initial work of the NIH Human Microbiome Project led to the conclusion that there is no core microbiome; that is, each individual has different microbes performing the same functions. Now, she noted, phase II of the Human Microbiome Project is conducting three cohort studies (i.e., of three different diseases) and analyzing both host and microbiome samples at a number of different "-omic" levels to get a better sense of the extent of interaction between the human host and its microbiome.

Janet King, workshop presenter, asked Donovan whether her finding that the gut microbiome in breastfed infants is more diverse than that of formula-fed infants may be due to the fact that breastmilk itself is diverse and, if so, what factors in breastmilk may be contributing. Donovan replied that much of the diversity in human breastmilk is diversity in the HMOs, which she said researchers have only begun to understand in the last 5-10 years. It is has been estimated that there are about 200 different HMOs, she noted, 10-12 of which constitute the majority of the milk HMOs in most women. She added that HMOs are the third most predominant component of breastmilk, after fat and lactose. Babies run on fat and sugar, she said, with all of these HMOs serving as the "fiber" of human breastmilk, which means they escape digestion in the upper end of the GI tract and end up in the lower GI tract.

Donovan reiterated that for her, what is fascinating about all of this recent work with the infant metagenome is that regardless of species, whether piglets, monkeys, or humans, feeding an artificial diet down-regulates gene expression overall. She cautioned, however, that the long-term implications of this finding are unclear, given that babies can be incredibly resilient. She suspects, however, that these early interactions may have adverse programming effects on long-term immune and metabolic outcomes.

Maha Tahiri, Food Forum member, asked Donovan whether there is evidence for interventions directed at the obesogenic programming effects of formula feeding versus breastfeeding. Donovan replied that at this point, she and her team have not identified such an intervention, but she mentioned an ongoing longitudinal cohort study of about 400 children that thus far has collected five stool samples for each child in the first year of life. The researchers will be following the children through the age of 5 years. Already they have seen distinct differences in growth trajectory among children with different microbiota. Donovan stressed the need for more prospective studies to determine whether differences in the microbiota influence early growth in infants and young children.

DIETARY INTERVENTIONS FOR HEALTHY AGING[11]

In the last presentation of day 1 of the workshop, de Cabo sought to translate to humans what has been learned from other species about the key pathways in aging. "Aging is a universal process," he said. Among all species, he noted, aging shows a sigmoidal effect (see Figure 4-7). He defined aging as the gradual change in structure and function of organisms that occurs with the passage of time, not as a result of disease or an accident. He stressed, however, that even among individuals who share the same culture or genes, the consequences of growing old (e.g., onset of first disease, longevity) may be very different among individuals because of gene–environment interactions and other factors.

Next, de Cabo echoed other speakers' emphasis on the fact that the world is aging and aging rapidly. For the first time in human history, he said, there are more people over age 65 than under age 5 (Population Division of the Department of Economic and Social Affairs of the United Nations Secretariat, 2005). He observed that the fastest-growing segments of today's human population are those aged 85 and older and aged 100 and older. He then described the almost exponential increase in the prevalence of disease with increasing age and emphasized that the major risk factor for the leading causes of death (heart disease, cancer, stroke, emphysema, pneumonia, diabetes, accidents, kidney disease, Alzheimer's) is aging itself, not obesity or some other factor. He argued that the mission of biomedical research is to increase the quality of life. Given that chronic diseases of the elderly are currently the main limitation on achieving an increase in the quality of life, he asserted, the major risk factor for all chronic diseases must be addressed, and that is aging itself.

---

[11]This section summarizes information presented by Dr. de Cabo.

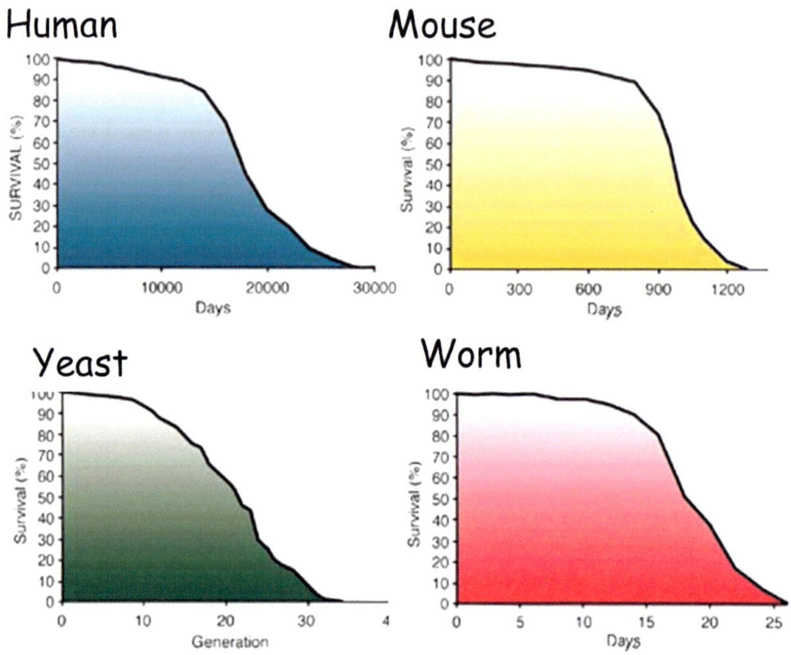

FIGURE 4-7 Survival (percentage of the population surviving) as a function of days (in humans, mice, and worms) or generations (in yeast).
SOURCE: Presented by R. de Cabo, September 13, 2016.

Caloric Restriction and Longevity

Can aging really be stopped? de Cabo asked. The short answer, he said, is "no," but in the laboratory, scientists have been able to alter both the onset and the progression of aging through interventions. He explained that over the past 500 years, the mean of the human lifespan has increased (i.e., people are living longer), and the sigmoidal shape of the survival curve has squared as a result of nutrition, the health care system, and public health (see Figure 4-8). He noted that this same shift has been replicated in the laboratory in animals by restricting daily total caloric intake (without malnutrition). Both mean and maximum lifespan have been shown to change (Weindruch and Sohal, 1997; Weindruch et al., 1979, 1986). According to de Cabo, caloric restriction has been shown to have an effect on lifespan in every species tested. Also important, in his opinion, it is not just age-related cancer but other age-related phenotypes, such as muscle structure and function (Everitt et al., 1985), that can be affected by caloric restriction.

"But there's always a catch," de Cabo continued. Namely, these lab-tested longevity interventions are lifelong interventions. It would be very difficult, he said, to convince people to eat for the rest of their lives 30-50 percent fewer calories every day. However, he explained, a growing understanding of some of the mechanisms that occur in response to caloric restriction has led to the identification of molecular targets (e.g., SIRT1, AMPK, mTOR, AKT/PKB) that potentially could be either activated or deactivated by different pharmacological compounds (de Cabo et al., 2014). He calls such compounds "caloric restriction mimetics." The goal, he explained, is to develop caloric restriction mimetics that have the same

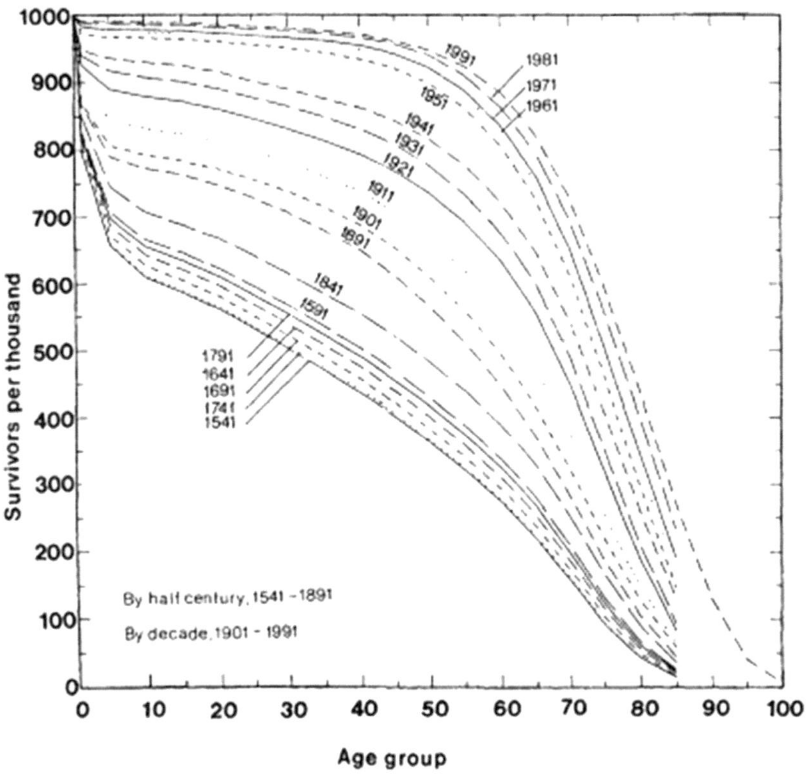

FIGURE 4-8 Change in the human survival curve over time, 1541-1991.
SOURCES: Presented by R. de Cabo, September 13, 2016. Kertzer and Laslett, 1995. Reprinted by permission from the University of California Press.

longevity and other beneficial effects of caloric restriction, but without its total reduction of caloric intake.

Caloric restriction mimetics have shown mixed results in the lab, however. For example, de Cabo noted that the effects of rapamycin have been shown to be substantially stronger in females than in males (Harrison et al., 2009; Miller et al., 2014), while the effects of acarbose have been shown to be strong in males but not in females (Harrison et al., 2014). After seeing these results, he went back to the literature and found that, although caloric restriction has been shown to have an effect on every species tested, there are in fact cases in which caloric restriction has not worked. It appears, he said, that many factors may influence the effects of caloric restriction, including not just sex but also genetic background, diet composition, and age.

To test the effects of some of these factors, de Cabo and colleagues designed an experiment with two common strains of mice, DBA and C57BL, and two levels of caloric restriction, 20 percent and 40 percent (Mitchell et al., 2016). Both strains showed reduced body weight over time at both levels of caloric restriction compared with mice on unrestricted diets, with the difference in body weight being dependent on both strain and sex. What was shocking, de Cabo said, was variation in survival by strain and sex (see Figure 4-9). For DBA females, there was no difference in survival between the 20 percent and 40 percent calorie-restricted groups, and de Cabo interpreted this result to mean that there was no added benefit for DBA females to restricting their diet by 40 percent rather than 20 percent. The same was true, more or less, with DBA males. In contrast, de Cabo reported, C57BL/6 females responded very differently to 20 percent versus 40 percent calorie restriction, with the former being associated with longer lifespan and the latter showing no difference from an unrestricted diet. In sum, he said, these results indicate that the response to caloric restriction in mice depended on strain (i.e., genetics), sex, and extent of caloric restriction.

In addition to caloric restriction mimetics, de Cabo mentioned several other similar strategies that have been proposed as ways to elicit the same effects as caloric restriction but without that form of restriction. These include time-restricted feeding, which involves providing food for very short periods of time; intermittent fasting, for example, eating one day, but not the next; and restriction of amino acids, such as methionine.

Caloric Restriction and the Brain

With respect to phenotypic effects of caloric restriction other than longevity, de Cabo remarked on the extensive mouse model work by Mark Mattson and colleagues showing a connection between energy restriction and the maintenance of optimal brain function and resistance to injury and disease. In one study, he reported, Mattson and colleagues conducted

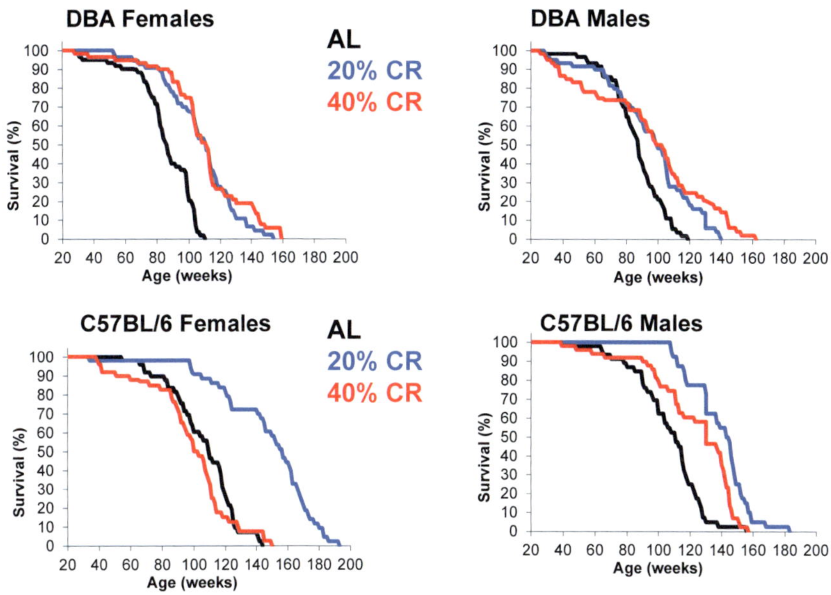

FIGURE 4-9 Survival curves for two strains of mice (DBA and C57BL/6), both females and males, on three different diets: regular diet (AL; black curves), 20 percent calorie-restricted diet (20 percent CR; blue curves), and 40 percent calorie-restricted diet (40 percent CR; red curves).
SOURCES: Presented by R. de Cabo, September 13, 2016. Reprinted from Mitchell et al., 2016, with permission from Elsevier.

a 3-month experiment in which they treated wild type and *db/db* (prone to diabetes) mice with either 40 percent caloric restriction or feeding every other day, both with and without exercise (running) (Stranaham et al., 2008, 2009). They found a drastic impact on dendritic spine density (in hippocampal neurons), which de Cabo described as markers of memory formation, and on BDNF levels in the hippocampus. Specifically, *db/db* mice who overate (i.e., were fed an ad libitum diet) exhibited reduced dendritic spine densities and BDNF levels compared with the control (normal-fed) mice. In both *db/db* and wild type mice, dietary restriction and running led to an increase in both dendritic spine densities and BDNF levels. In another study cited by de Cabo, using a mouse model of Alzheimer's disease (i.e., in which the mice overexpress three proteins that have been associated with Alzheimer's), caloric restriction led to an improvement in learning and retention of memory (Halagappa et al., 2007).

The Future of Caloric Restriction in Humans

In summary, de Cabo stated that the lifespan of most species studied can be extended by caloric restriction. This awareness, he said, has led to the identification of several underlying molecular pathways (e.g., IGF, sirtuins, mTOR), which in turn has led to the search for molecules that can target those pathways. To date, he noted, about 15 such molecules have been identified. He reiterated that there are a growing number of nonmolecular caloric restriction strategies as well (e.g., intermittent fasting, restricted feeding). He recalled that when he started research in this area in 2000, there was only one way to extend lifespan nongenetically, and that was caloric restriction. With continued research on the mechanisms of caloric restriction and the basic biology of aging, he predicts future success in the translation of these results to humans.

Meanwhile, de Cabo suggested that many of these interventions could also be translated to improve what he referred to as human "healthspan." Rapamycin, for example, has been shown in mice to stop skin tumors (Checkley et al., 2011) and the deposition of amyloid plaques (Caccamo et al., 2010). Importantly, de Cabo said, some of these findings have already been translated to humans. He cited one study in which administration of an analogue of rapamycin led to an improved response to vaccination in elderly individuals (i.e., via mTOR inhibition [Mannick et al., 2014]). In other work, Brandhorst and colleagues (2015) showed that periodic short-term fasting can protect against carcinogenesis and other risk factors of aging.

In conclusion, de Cabo believes that in the future, more tools will be available with which to identify for whom, when, and how longevity interventions can or should be applied. He emphasized the need to develop predictive biomarkers for healthy aging and longevity for use in future work.

5

Moving Forward

On the second day of the workshop, in Session 4, moderated by Johanna Dwyer, senior nutrition scientist, Office of Dietary Supplements (ODS), National Institutes of Health (NIH), the focus of discussion shifted to the future and ways to promote healthy aging. First, David Reuben, director, Multicampus Program in Geriatric Medicine and Gerontology, and chief, Division of Geriatrics, University of California, Los Angeles (UCLA), provided an overview of results from observational studies and clinical trials on three diets and their effects on health in older individuals: (1) the Mediterranean diet, (2) the DASH (Dietary Approaches to Stop Hypertension) diet, and (3) the MIND (Mediterranean-DASH Intervention for Neurodegenerative Delay) diet. Next, Eve Stoody, lead nutritionist of nutrition guidance, Center for Nutrition Policy and Promotion (CNPP), U.S. Department of Agriculture (USDA), provided an overview of the *2015-2020 Dietary Guidelines for Americans* (DGA), discussed dietary intake across the lifespan, and highlighted opportunities for the future. Finally, Timothy Morck, president and founder, Spectrum Nutrition LLC, and Douglas "Duffy" MacKay, senior vice president, scientific and regulatory affairs, Council for Responsible Nutrition (CRN), discussed the role of the food industry in supporting healthy aging.

NUTRITION TO PROMOTE HEALTHY AGING[1]

Based on his experience working with geriatric patients, Reuben emphasized the heterogeneity of the older population with respect not only to health but also to risks associated with malnutrition (e.g., being heavier may actually be beneficial for some older individuals; see the summary of Gordon Jensen's presentation in Chapter 3), as well as barriers to good nutrition (e.g., loss of teeth, chronic diseases with dietary restrictions, medications that interfere with appetite).

Focusing on barriers to good nutrition, Reuben mentioned that some activities of daily living and instrumental activities of daily living, such as going shopping and feeding oneself, become more difficult as one grows older and frailer, and loss of teeth makes it difficult to eat (see the summary of Athena Papas's presentation in Chapter 4). As an example of a chronic disease associated with dietary restriction, he mentioned a patient of his with kidney disease whose potassium keeps rising and who is not eating much. He said he does not want to restrict her dietary intake given that she is already not eating much. "But she really can't eat foods containing potassium," he said, "or else she's going to wind up in the hospital." Finally, although medications administered to older adults occasionally cause weight gain, he observed, most interfere with appetite.

Additionally, Reuben emphasized variation in nutritional health among subpopulations. While healthier older people may have the same nutritional needs they had in mid-life, many others have chronic diseases or are frail and have limited life expectancy. Finally, he noted, whether older adults live in the community, an assisted living facility, or a nursing home can also affect their nutritional health, as can the extent to which individuals in any of these environments go in and out of hospitals. The nutritional requirements of each of these populations in each of these environments are different, he observed.

Three Diets and Their Effects on Health in Older Individuals

The majority of Reuben's presentation revolved around results from observational studies and clinical trials on three diets and their effects on health in older individuals: (1) the Mediterranean diet, (2) the DASH diet, and (3) the MIND diet. He began by describing each of these diets. He noted that while the Mediterranean and DASH diets have much in common, there are some differences. Whereas the DASH diet recommends high intake of low-fat dairy, for example, the Mediterranean diet recommends low intake of full-fat dairy. Fish is classified differently in the two diets as

[1]This section summarizes information presented by Dr. Reuben.

well (the DASH diet recommends low fish intake, whereas the Mediterranean diet recommends high fish intake). But by and large, Reuben said, the two diets share many of the same principles. The MIND diet, which bills itself as a blend of the DASH and Mediterranean diets, is operationalized a little differently, he noted, with more nuts and berries and some foods in the DASH and Mediterranean diets not being included.

Results from Observational Studies

Reuben reported that most observational studies of these three diets have been cohort studies that have relied on dietary questionnaires, food frequencies, and similar tools. For the Mediterranean and DASH diets, he said, observational data have shown significant decreases in several adverse health outcomes, including cardiovascular disease (9 percent reduction); cancer (with measured effects varying from 6 to 10 percent overall, based on two separate meta-analyses, to a 14 percent reduction for colorectal, 4 percent for prostate, and 56 percent for pharyngeal/esophageal cancer); overall mortality (9 percent reduction); and Parkinson's and Alzheimer's diseases (13 percent reduction) (Schwingshackl and Hoffman, 2014; Sofi et al., 2008). He added that a number of other studies have shown multiple effects of these diets on a range of other outcomes, from chronic kidney disease to depression.

Reuben reported that observational data for the MIND diet have shown less decline in several cognitive outcomes relative to the other two diets, based on a 4.7-year cohort study on a group of individuals at risk for dementia (Morris et al., 2015). These individuals were not prescribed a MIND diet, he explained; rather, they followed one. Results at 4.7 years showed less decline in global, episodic, semantic, and working memory; perceptual speed; and perceptual organization. Most impressively, in Reuben's opinion, the MIND dieters were less likely to develop Alzheimer's disease at 4.5 years (Morris et al., 2015).

Results from Clinical Trials

According to Reuben, clinical trial data on these diets have similarly shown significant reductions in adverse health outcomes. The PREDIMED study of the Mediterranean and DASH diets is probably the most "famous" clinical trial of any of these diets, he remarked. Individuals aged 55-80 were randomized into three arms: (1) Mediterranean diet plus extra virgin olive oil, (2) Mediterranean diet plus mixed nuts, and (3) regular diet with reduced dietary fat (the control). The primary outcome was a composite of myocardial infarction, stroke, and cardiovascular death at 4.8 years post-study. Results showed a 28-30 percent reduction in this primary outcome in the two experimental arms relative to the control group (Estruch et al., 2013). Reuben noted that the effect size was the same among young older persons (less than 70) and old older persons (70 and above). He also cited data from other clinical trials showing that the DASH diet lowered blood pressure and cholesterol as well (Siervo et al., 2015).

Reuben reported on a secondary analysis of PREDIMED data focused on cognition outcomes, which showed that the same interventions were also associated with higher cognitive functioning at 6.5 years poststudy (specifically, higher Mini Mental State Examination [MMSE] and Clock-Drawing Test scores) (Martínez-Lapiscina et al., 2013). Additionally, he noted, a short-term randomized clinical trial of the DASH diet showed greater psychomotor skills at 4 months (Smith et al., 2010).

Nutritional Supplements and Disease Outcomes in Older Individuals

Next, Reuben summarized some of what is known about the relationship between nutritional supplements and disease outcomes in older individuals.

Recommendations for Vitamin D and Calcium Supplementation

Reuben cited conflicting recommendations with respect to vitamin D and calcium supplementation. The U.S. Preventive Services Task Force (USPSTF) makes no recommendation. (Nor does the USPSTF make any recommendations for any vitamin, mineral, or multivitamin supplements to prevent heart disease, or for beta carotene or vitamin E.) The Institute of Medicine (IOM, 2011), by contrast, recommended 800 international units of vitamin D3 daily and 1,200 mg of calcium daily for individuals aged 71 and older. Reuben noted that the IOM recommendation is the more commonly cited one.

Evidence on the Effects of Calcium Supplementation

Reuben explained that the controversy over calcium supplementation revolves around its actual effects when used as a supplement, as opposed to increasing calcium intake through the diet, which he noted may have different effects. Data from the Women's Health Initiative showed no increased risk for either heart attack or stroke with calcium supplementation (Hsia et al., 2007), he said. However, a meta-analysis did show a slightly increased risk, with a relative risk (RR) of 1.27 for calcium alone and an RR of 1.24 when calcium supplementation was combined with vitamin D (Bolland et al., 2010, 2011).

In August 2016, Reuben continued, a small observational study conducted in Europe was published in *Neurology*. An odds ratio (OR) of 2.10 for dementia was reported among individuals taking calcium supplements, and the OR for stroke-related dementia was 4.4 and 6.77 among individuals with a history of stroke, compared with women not receiving supplementation (Kern et al., 2016).

Evidence on the Effects of Multivitamins

Turning to the effects of multivitamins, Reuben reported that observational data from the Women's Health Initiative in postmenopausal women showed no benefit or protective effect on breast, colorectal, endometrial, lung, or ovarian cancers; myocardial infarction; venous thromboembolism; or mortality (Mursu et al., 2011). In middle-aged men, he observed, a meta-analysis of clinical trial data indicated that multivitamins have not been shown to decrease cardiovascular disease or mortality, but have been shown to be associated with a small reduction in total cancer risk (Macpherson et al., 2013). Additionally, he said, several clinical trials conducted in nursing homes or outpatient settings have shown no benefit of multivitamins in reducing infections.

Evidence from the AREDS2 Trial

Reuben cited results from the AREDS2 trial, which came out in 2015, showing no benefit of fatty acids (docosahexaenoic acid [DHA] and eicosapentaenoic acid [EPA]), antioxidants (lutein and zeaxanthin), or zinc supplements with respect to cognitive decline (Chew et al., 2015). He explained that this study was not focused on health but on vision and prevention of the progression of macular degeneration. While conducting the study, however, the researchers ran a large set of cognitive tests. Unfortunately, in Reuben's opinion, "any way you sliced it," the results of the cognitive tests showed no improvement from these supplements.

QUESTIONS FOR THE FIELD

Finally, Reuben raised several questions for the field:

- How can the DGA that apply to older persons be promoted and included in prevention and health care settings? Reuben observed that "almost nothing" is going on in health care settings with respect to advising older adults on nutrition.
- How can the barriers to good nutrition that are unique to older persons be overcome? Reuben referred to his earlier description of the various settings and populations of older adults. He mentioned

some nursing homes that will not even accept patients without gastrostomy tubes because of the cost of labor required to feed people.

- Is evidence for the Mediterranean and DASH diets compelling enough for these diets to be implemented widely, and if so, what would be the best strategy? Reuben suspects that very few people are aware of these diets and that most people would probably guess they are weight-loss strategies.
- What can be recommended for people for whom these diets would not be appropriate (i.e., those whose life expectancy is 3-5 years or less, who are extremely frail, or who have multiple chronic diseases)?
- What is the appropriate stance on multivitamins and other nutritional supplements for which evidence of benefit does not exist? Reuben remarked that many of his patients take as many nutritional supplements as they do medications. In his opinion, an enormous amount of money is being spent on nutritional supplements with no benefit.
- When, if ever, is it reasonable to stop preventive nutritional measures? Reuben said he has a number of patients who have "graduated" into the category of "eat whatever you want." The greater issue for them is not nutrition, but consuming any calories at all.
- What more needs to be known? What would the research agenda be for older people and nutrition? What kinds of studies need to be done in these populations with respect not only to creating new knowledge but also to applying what is known? Reuben suspects that some areas are ready for implementation science, while others would benefit from more epidemiological and clinical trial data.

QUESTIONS FROM THE AUDIENCE

Following his talk, Reuben fielded questions from the audience on a range of topics. He was asked to elaborate on how much evidence exists to indicate when preventive nutrition measures should be stopped. In his opinion, this frame of thinking needs to shift when an individual's remaining time is no longer indefinite. Up to that point, he said, while it is known that certain foods are better than others, this knowledge is not very precise. That said, there is a knowledge base on preventive nutrition measures, and it is an increasingly good one in his opinion. He believes the field has gotten closer to conducting a public education campaign (e.g., so that people know about the Mediterranean and DASH diets) and implementing these interventions. Moreover, he suggested, now is a good time to do this, as people are beginning to pay attention to nutrition.

When asked whether the benefits of the Mediterranean and DASH diets derive from what those diets add or what they reduce, Reuben replied that he thinks reducing red meats and high-fat foods is probably what matters most. Based on his own living as a vegetarian, he commented on how difficult it can be to eat a vegetarian diet. He commented that he has had to walk out of restaurants because of the lack of menu items he would eat.

There was some discussion around supplements. Simin Meydani, workshop participant, remarked that meta-analysis results have shown that supplementation with vitamin E below 200 mg/day not only causes no harm but may have some benefit in lowering mortality. She suggested that perhaps the recommendation for vitamin E supplementation should be dose-dependent. Reuben agreed that finding an appropriate dose for some of these supplements may involve "threading the needle." He mentioned a study showing that supplemental vitamin E doses of 1,000 mg twice daily slowed cognitive decline.

When asked about the multiple medicines being prescribed for older adults, Reuben suggested that the challenge is not only that many medicines interact with each other but also that taking that many pills per day is difficult. Remembering to take 8, 10, or 12 different medicines every day, for example, can be challenging.

MacKay remarked that, while he appreciated looking at supplements through the lens of reducing disease risk, he believes that not underscoring the importance of just meeting targeted nutrient intakes independently of disease prevention is like "throwing the baby out with the bathwater." He added that in his opinion, results of the Physicians Health Study II, which showed a statistically significant 8 percent reduction in total cancer associated with taking a daily multivitamin, had been downplayed. Reuben replied that his intention was not to criticize the supplement industry. He said he often recommends supplements and acknowledged that some people are not getting enough of their basic vitamins from their diet and would benefit from a multivitamin. On the other hand, he believes that people who have a good diet probably get all the vitamins and minerals they need from their diet.

The last question was on recommendations for research, education, and communication to help promote healthy aging through nutrition. Reuben replied that doctors like to prescribe pills. "It is incredibly gratifying," he said. He suggested that this same approach be considered for nutrition; that is, physicians should be able to prescribe certain types of diets to their patients, who would then get these prescriptions filled not by a pharmacist but by a nutritionist. Importantly, he said, this would have to happen at the level of the primary care physician. If primary care physicians do not have respect for good nutrition and are unaware of what it can do for a patient, he argued, they are not going to prescribe a certain type of diet—they are going to prescribe a medicine. The problem starts, in his opinion, in medical education. He described the culture, or mindset, of physicians as different from that of those who teach nutrition. Moderator Johanna Dwyer added, "And we must not forget the nurses."

PATTERNS OF DIETARY INTAKE ACROSS THE LIFESPAN AND OPPORTUNITIES TO SUPPORT HEALTHY AGING[2]

Stoody emphasized that lifespan is at the core of the 2015-2020 DGA (HHS and USDA, 2015). The U.S. Department of Health and Human Services (HHS) and USDA, she reported, have been working together since 1980 to release new editions of the DGA every 5 years. The 2015-2020 edition was released in January 2016. Stoody explained that the current edition includes 5 guidelines and 13 recommendations and is 144 pages long. As in past editions, she added, it continues to refer to individual components of the diet, but with an increased focus on dietary patterns as a whole and their adaptability based on age, sex, physical activity level, preferences, and other factors. She quoted from Chapter 1 of the guidelines (HHS and USDA, 2015, p. 14): "The goal of the *Dietary Guidelines* is for individuals throughout all stages of the lifespan to have eating patterns that promote overall health and help prevent chronic disease." Additionally, she noted, the first of the five guidelines is to "follow a healthy eating pattern across the lifespan."

A key recommendation of the 2015-2020 DGA, Stoody pointed out, is to follow a healthy eating pattern that accounts for all food and beverages within an appropriate calorie level. The guidelines define a healthy pattern as one that includes a variety of vegetables from all subgroups (dark green, red and orange, legumes [beans and peas], starchy, and other); fruits, especially whole fruits; grains, at least half of which are whole grains; fat-free or low-fat dairy, including milk, yogurt, cheese, and fortified soy beverages; a variety of protein foods, including seafood, lean meats and poultry, eggs, legumes (beans and peas), nuts and seeds, and soy products; and oils. Additionally, a healthy pattern limits saturated and trans fats, added sugars, and sodium. There are some specific quantitative recommendations for components of the diet that should be limited, Stoody noted: to consume less than 10 percent of calories per day from added sugars; to consume less than 10 percent of calories per day from saturated fats; to consume less than 2,300 mg per day of sodium (or the age-appropriate dietary reference tolerable upper intake level); and, if alcohol is consumed, to consume it in moderation (up to one drink per day for women and up to two drinks per day for men), and only if one is an adult of legal drinking age.

[2]This section summarizes information presented by Dr. Stoody.

Meeting the DGA Recommendations: Variation Across the Lifespan

"So how are we doing in meeting these recommendations?" Stoody asked. Based on measures of the Healthy Eating Index (HEI) over the last several cycles of the National Health and Nutrition Examination Survey (NHANES),[3] among individuals aged 2 years and older, average HEI scores had reached only 57.8 (with a maximum score being 100) by 2009-2010 (see Figure 5-1). "There is obviously a lot of room for improvement," Stoody said. Breaking these HEI data down by age group, she noted, reveals some variability among those aged 2-17, 18-64, and 65 and older (see Figure 5-2).

In addition to looking at measures of the total diet (i.e., HEI), Stoody suggested examining individual components of the diet separately and the percentage of the U.S. population aged 1 year and older at, above, or below each dietary goal or limit (see Figure 5-3). Again, she observed, a large percentage of the American population does not meet these recommendations. As an example, she pointed out that almost 90 percent of the population fails to meet the recommendation for vegetables. The percentage of the population meeting the recommendation for fruit is slightly better. But about 70 percent of the population is not meeting the recommended limits for added sugars and saturated fats, and an even greater percentage are not meeting the recommended limits for sodium.

Stoody then considered several selected dietary components separately (i.e., vegetables, fruits, dairy, total grains, protein foods, sodium, added sugars, and saturated fats). She examined average daily intakes of these components across the lifespan for both sexes and compared these with recommended intakes (see Figure 5-4). She emphasized that at some stages of the lifespan, certain components of the diet are of greater concern relative to other stages of the lifespan. For example, she pointed out, average intakes for the age group 1-3 years generally fall either within or near the recommended ranges for most food components. In adolescence (ages 14-18), in contrast, vegetable and fruit intake is low for both females and males, dairy intake is particularly low for females, and intake of added sugars is high for both females and males. Among older adults (age 71 and above), while vegetable and fruit intakes are still low, the gap between these intakes and recommended levels is not as great as it is among younger individuals, and intakes of total grains and protein are near recommended levels. And added sugars and sodium are not as great a concern as with younger age groups.

In summary, Stoody said, most Americans need to shift their dietary

[3]The NHANES is a repeated cross-sectional survey conducted annually that provides population-level estimates of dietary intake and trends.

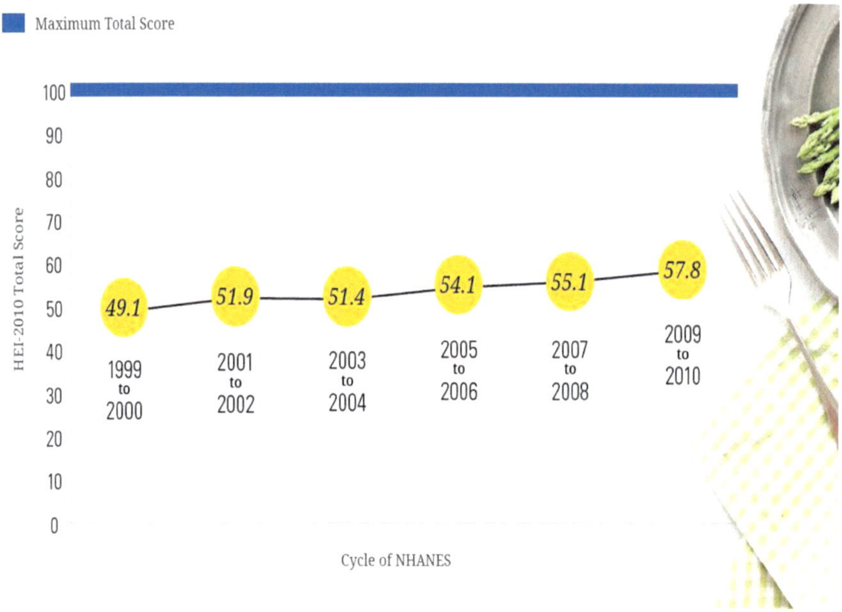

FIGURE 5-1 Average Healthy Eating Index (HEI) scores of the U.S. population, aged 2 years and older, as a function of the National Health and Nutrition Examination Survey (NHANES) cycle, 1999-2000 to 2009-2010.
SOURCES: Presented by E. Stoody, September 14, 2016. HHS and USDA, 2015.

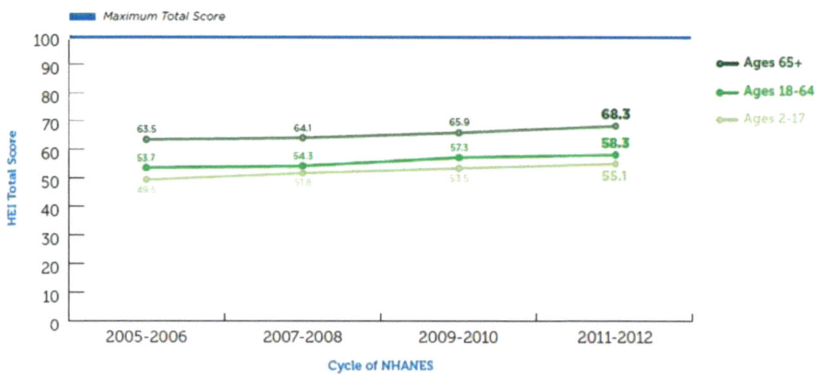

FIGURE 5-2 Average Healthy Eating Index (HEI) scores of the U.S. population as a function of the National Health and Nutrition Examination Survey (NHANES) cycle, 2005-2006 to 2011-2012, by age group.
SOURCES: Presented by E. Stoody, September 14, 2016. USDA, 2017.

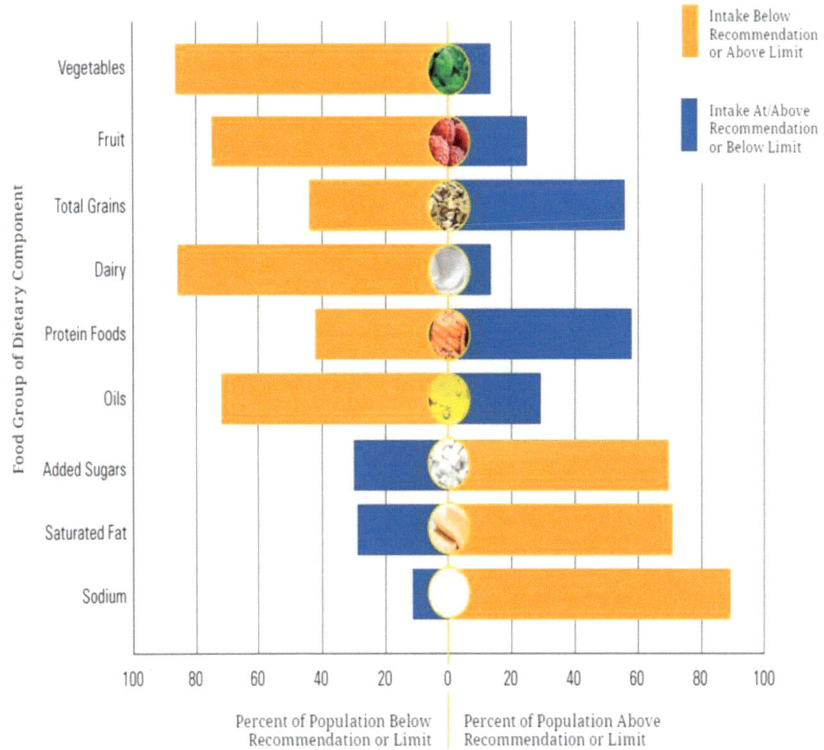

FIGURE 5-3 Percentage of the U.S. population aged 1 year and older who are below, at, or above recommended minimums or limits for certain food groups and other dietary components.
SOURCES: Presented by E. Stoody, September 14, 2016. HHS and USDA, 2015.

intakes to achieve healthy eating patterns. She noted that while some of these needed shifts are minor and can be accomplished by making simple substitutions, others will require greater effort to accomplish. Finally, young children and older Americans are generally closer to the recommendations relative to adolescents and young adults.

The Future of the DGA

With respect to opportunities for future work, Stoody emphasized three areas: (1) implementation of the current DGA, (2) recommendations in future DGA, and (3) future research.

Regarding implementation of the DGA, Stoody referenced the graph

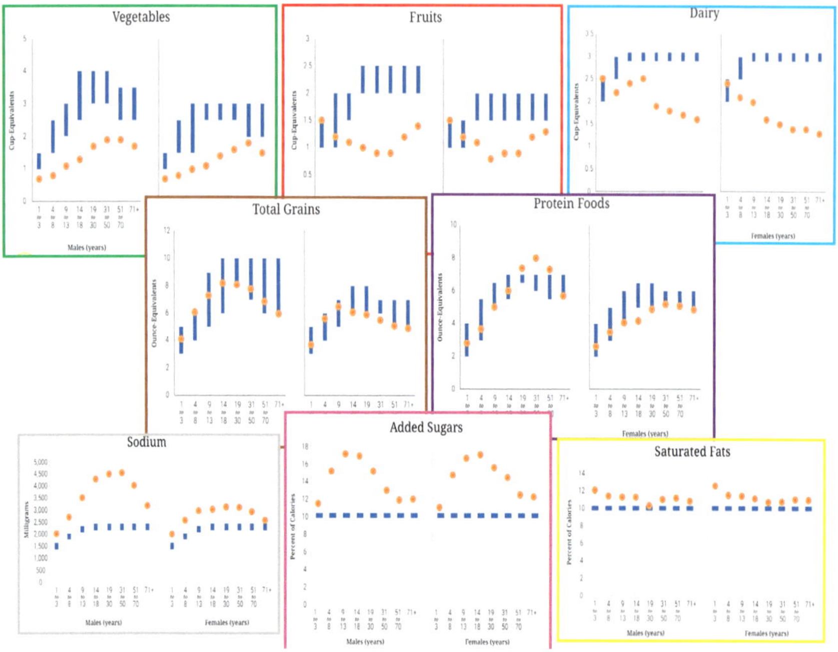

FIGURE 5-4 Average daily intakes (yellow dots) compared with recommended intake ranges (blue bars) for selected food groups and other dietary components, by age, for both males (the left graph of each pair) and females (the right graph of each pair).
SOURCES: Presented by E. Stoody, September 14, 2016. HHS and USDA, 2015.

in Figure 5-2, which shows HEI trends over time for three different age groups, and suggested that improving the intakes of young children and maintaining those intakes as children grow into adolescence could result in healthy eating patterns across the lifespan. The question, though, is how. Stoody recalled some discussion from the previous day around the reality that simply telling people they need to eat healthier is not working. In her opinion, a much bigger conversation is necessary. As the DGA state, "Everyone has a role in helping to create and support healthy eating patterns in multiple settings nationwide, from home to school to work to communities." Stoody noted that the DGA include a socioecological model that covers multiple areas in which change can be supported not just at the individual level but also among sectors, settings, and different social and cultural values and norms.

One of the ways in which change is supported through the federal government, Stoody continued, is through MyPlate. She remarked that a number of materials are available through ChooseMyPlate.gov to support healthy eating, including tailored, audience-specific resources for different stages of life (i.e., preschoolers, youth, older individuals). She mentioned the considerable collaborative work on promoting MyPlate, including an initiative in collaboration with the National Institute on Aging to create materials such as "10 healthy eating tips for people age 65+."[4] She noted that the National Institute on Aging's Go4Life program has additional materials to help support healthy eating in specific settings beyond individual behavior change.

With respect to the future 2020-2025 DGA, Stoody stated that while the DGA have traditionally included recommendations for Americans aged 2 years and older, there has been a growing demand to expand the DGA to cover the population aged 0-24 months. Indeed, she noted, the Agricultural Act of 2014 mandated that the 2020-2025 DGA include dietary guidance for this youngest population, as well as women who are pregnant. For Stoody, this expansion of the DGA raises the question of whether other stages of life warrant more comprehensive guidance, and whether older adults are one of those stages. The current and previous guidelines do apply to older adults generally, she acknowledged, and since 1980, the guidelines have included specific guidance for older individuals (see Figure 5-5). But again, she asked, "Should there be more? Should there be some sort of comprehensive guidance?" In her opinion, this is a conversation that should be taking place.

With respect to future research, Stoody reiterated that the current edition of the DGA is focused on dietary patterns, informed by an evidence base of those patterns in relation to various health outcomes, including cardiovascular disease, body weight, type 2 diabetes, certain types of cancer, bone health, depression, and dementia/cognitive impairment/Alzheimer's disease. In general, however, she believes more evidence is needed across the lifespan. She observed that most of the studies on dietary patterns in the evidence base for the 2015-2020 DGA included subjects who were aged 50 and older (mean age) at baseline and who were followed for approximately 10 years. There is still a gap, she asserted, in understanding how dietary patterns across the *entire* lifespan contribute to healthy aging. Additionally, she suggested, improved methods are needed for assessing dietary patterns more comprehensively, precisely, and with standardization so that investigators can better define habitual food intake in populations. She noted that some of this work is under way. She also called for stronger methodological

[4]See https://www.nia.nih.gov/health/publication/choosing-healthy-meals-you-get-older (accessed January 18, 2017).

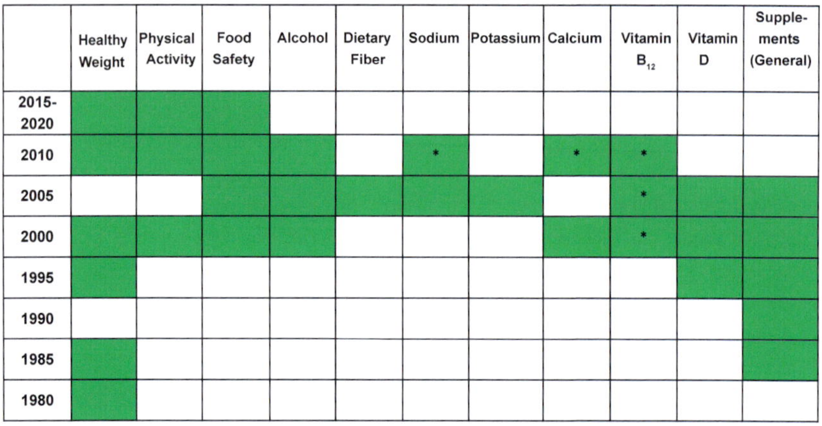

FIGURE 5-5 Areas in the *2015-2020 Dietary Guidelines for Americans* (DGA) in which guidance includes specific statements focused on older individuals.
NOTES: The recommendations of the DGA apply generally to older individuals, but there are cases in which specific statements have focused on this population. * Indicates that these topics are covered for adults aged 50/51 and older.
SOURCE: Presented by E. Stoody, September 14, 2016.

designs—for example, longer duration of follow-up, assessment of dietary intake at multiple time points over the course of a study, and cohort studies that start earlier in life and that capture dietary patterns contributing to health outcomes later in life.

DISCUSSION WITH THE AUDIENCE

In the discussion following Stoody's presentation, her observation that the gap between recommended and actual intakes was smallest for children elicited a comment from Wendy Johnson-Askew about the difference between this finding and that of Gerber's Feeding Infants and Toddlers Study (FITS) regarding fruit and vegetable intake in infants and toddlers—namely, that this intake is low, particularly for vegetables. In contrast to results presented by Stoody, she observed, FITS data have shown that most young children are not consuming a discrete vegetable serving on any day. In fact, she noted, it was these results from the 2008 FITS study that influenced changes to the Special Supplemental Nutrition Program for Women, Infants, and Children (WIC) food package. Now, Gerber is struggling to find "stealth" ways to provide more vegetables to babies and toddlers. Johnson-Askew asked whether there were methodological differences between FITS and the studies that yielded the results Stoody had shared and what data sources informed Stoody's analysis. Stoody responded that the NHANES data on fruit and vegetable intake used to inform the analysis she had shared included mixed dishes (for vegetables) and 100 percent fruit juice (for fruits). Johnson-Askew added that in fact, with infants' high saturated fat and sodium intakes, their diets (based on FITS data) actually mimic those of adults. She referred to a recent U.S. Centers for Disease Control and Prevention (CDC) study, published in *Pediatrics*, that produced results very similar to those of FITS. She noted that the CDC study was longitudinal, and showed that eating patterns established in early childhood lasted through the age of 6. She said that, based on what has been observed with NHANES adult data, she suspects these same early eating patterns track all the way through adulthood.

Johnson-Askew's comments prompted an audience member to comment on vegetable intake as being problematic across the lifespan. In this audience member's opinion, people do not like the taste of vegetables (e.g., they detect the bitterness or do not like the smell of broccoli when it is cooked). It is not enough, she said, to tell people to eat their vegetables. The challenge, in her opinion, is to incorporate vegetables into dishes in a way that creates flavor profiles people are willing to embrace. Stoody replied that another analysis conducted for the 2015-2020 DGA revealed that the top source of calories was mixed dishes. She observed that incorporating vegetables into these mixed dishes already being consumed may be a strategy for increasing vegetable consumption.

Johanna Dwyer commented on the fact that most people over age 75 or 80 have one or two chronic conditions and that the majority of these people take dietary supplements. She suspects that about half of these older adults also take multivitamins. She observed that some of the assumptions underlying dietary guidance for very old adults appear to be very different from those for younger adults and wondered whether it might be time to develop DGA for adults aged 75 and older. Stoody agreed that it is worth talking about whether any stages of life warrant more comprehensive coverage for which the evidence base exists. She reiterated that older adults might be one of those stages.

Finally, regarding the gaps between recommended and actual intake levels, not just for fruits and vegetables but for all food groups, there was some discussion around the reality that many consumers do not understand some basic concepts in nutrition. Thus while, in one audience member's opinion, ChooseMyPlate provides a great visual, a gap remains in consumers' understanding of what that visual actually means. Many consumers do not understand the concept of cup-equivalent, or whole grain cup-equivalent, for example. Stoody agreed and added that the messages that need to be communicated depend on the age group of the audience. She noted that the National Institute on Aging, for example, communicates about cup-equivalents in a way that is appropriate for older adults. Adding to the confusion, she observed, is that the population has to contend with different messages being communicated from different sources about what constitutes a healthy diet. She encouraged a more collective voice across the nutrition community and communication through a more collaborative lens.

SUPPORTING HEALTHY AGING ACROSS THE LIFESPAN: THE ROLE OF THE FOOD INDUSTRY[5]

What Constitutes the Food Industry?

In the first of two presentations on the role of the food industry in promoting healthy aging, Morck elaborated on the industry's complexity. He began by asking, "What constitutes the food industry?" He emphasized the expansiveness of the industry and described its many components, each of which is focused on its own categorical products.

First, Morck explained, are the commodity producers (i.e., producers of raw components), including a "farm fresh" organic component that Morck noted is becoming very popular. Next are the processed/packaged foods, including different types of meal components (e.g., frozen peas, breakfast cereal, pasta), as well as sauces, spreads, dressings, and condiments. These also include prepared dairy products (e.g., yogurt, cheese). Also within this component of the food industry are ingredient suppliers. They are the ones, Morck said, that are capitalizing on bioactives and finding new opportunities to enrich foods in ways, for example, that may influence the microbiome. Another component is the composite meal producers and suppliers. Composite meals include multicomponent entrees, pizzas, and handheld and other "simpler" meals. Yet another component is snacks and desserts, which include salty snacks, confections, and baked and frozen desserts (e.g., ice cream). The beverage component of the food industry includes soft drinks, water, tea, coffee, juices, alcoholic beverages, sports drinks, energy drinks, and fortified beverages. Other food industry components include the makers of specially formulated nutritional products (e.g., infant formula), foods with limited or omitted nutrients or components (e.g., gluten-free products), dietary supplements, and medical foods (i.e., foods for patients with distinctive nutrient requirements that cannot be met by altering the diet alone).

Yet another entirely different dimension of the food industry and food intake, Morck continued, is out-of-home food consumption, including

[5]This section summarizes information presented by Dr. Morck.

quick-serve restaurants, sit-down restaurants, and take-away. Relative to other components, this is a component of the food industry over which consumers have much less control in terms of menu choices, he observed. While this situation is beginning to change, he suggested, with some disclosures about calories and some discussion around sodium levels, this area of food intake remains, in his opinion, one that is particularly difficult to manage. The restaurant industry is a $783 billion industry, he noted, accounting for close to 50 percent of food dollars being spent, compared with 25 percent in 1955.

Finally, Morck explained, also out-of-home is the food service component of the food industry. This component includes hospitals; schools; prisons; cafeterias; workplace food services; vending services; and government program suppliers, including school lunch programs, the Supplemental Nutrition Assistance Program (SNAP), WIC, and the military.

Given this expansiveness, Morck suggested, when the question is raised of what the food industry contributes to healthy aging, the question really is what consumers are choosing from this panoply of options to meet their own needs. That said, he asserted, over the past 5-10 years, the food industry has in fact made significant progress toward supporting healthy eating—for example, by reducing sugar, fat, and calories and eliminating trans fat from the food supply. He described how the production and promotion of healthier foods is one of several public commitments endorsed by food company members of the Grocery Manufacturers Association (GMA), and one for which they are held publicly accountable. GMA is one of the major trade associations of the food industry, he explained.

Drivers That Impact the Food Industry, Support the Food Industry Requires, and What the Food Industry Can Do to Support Healthy Aging

Eliciting the support of the food industry in healthy aging, Morck continued, requires understanding the drivers that impact the industry. First, he emphasized, the food industry sells only products that people buy. It is driven by consumer purchases, with repeat sales based on consumer satisfaction being required for success. Morck referred to the Campbell Soup Company's initial introduction of reduced-sodium soups as an example of a product change that consumers did not like, forcing the company to dial back its aggressive sodium reduction targets. Second, he observed that people typically do not eat just to fulfill a physiological requirement. Rather, they eat for social, emotional, and other reasons as well, with different people turning to different foods for these purposes. Cost, variety, ethnicity, and availability also drive the diversity of product offerings. Third, Morck said, the industry is governed by regulatory guidelines on marketing, communications, nutrition labeling, and claims. As an example, he mentioned guidelines for marketing and communicating to children in particular. Finally, he explained, the industry is driven by its overarching commitment to food safety and quality and is constantly striving to improve manufacturing efficiency to keep costs down (i.e., the greater the efficiency, the lower the cost). He added that the food industry is also publicly embracing an increased commitment to incorporating sustainable practices across the supply chain.

According to Morck, the food industry's provision of nutritional support for healthy aging requires, first, compelling research outcomes with practical applications. He explained that the industry is happy to develop products consistent with the research if it can then communicate to consumers the outcomes of that research and what they can expect from consuming those products. He also called for new tools for identifying and targeting susceptible individuals for personalized recommendations to promote "their" healthy aging, with respect, for example, to their health/disease state, microbiota, or genetic predisposition. He called as well for a cooperative and collaborative regulatory agency to approve validated claims for products when appropriate data are provided, endorsement of evidence-based nutrition concepts by physicians and regulators when these concepts are shown to be cost-effective and therapeutic for patients, and the effective use of social media and technology to bring positive messages about health improvement to consumers.

Currently, Morck continued, health claims approved by the U.S. Food and Drug Administration (FDA) represent one means of informing consumers how consumption of certain levels of foods that contribute certain amounts of nutrients may help prevent and reduce the risk of future chronic disease. There are about 18 of these health claims, he noted. Qualified health claims are what he described as more "aggressive" because the strength of the evidence required is not as conclusive as that required for unqualified claims, with this uncertainty having to be disclosed along with potential benefit. According to Morck, the complexity of the language required for qualified health claims is so "obtuse," and not "consumer-friendly," that companies are reluctant to use it on their packaging.

Health claims aside, Morck reiterated that the food industry has in fact made significant progress toward supporting healthy eating by reducing sugar, fat, and calories and eliminating trans fat from the food supply. Additionally, the industry has added dietary fiber, mainly through whole grains in flour and soluble fiber in drinks; increased protein, Omega-3 fatty acids, probiotics, iron, and antioxidant vitamins; developed early-stage formulations to hydrolyze proteins and reduce the allergic potential for infants allergic to cow's milk; and provided medical foods for patients unable to consume normal foods.

Almost all of the large food industry companies are partners in the

Healthy Weight Commitment Foundation, according to Morck. This is not "just a food program," he stressed. The foundation works with communities, including educators and coaches, toward the goal of removing 1.5 trillion calories from the food supply. At last calculation, Morck reported, 6.4 trillion calories had been removed.

In summary, Morck said, the food industry can promote and support research that establishes links between nutrition and healthy aging at all stages of life. He remarked that, although it is becoming more difficult for industry to partner with academia because of perceptions of industry-funded research, industry does fund academic research. He stressed that testing hypotheses through appropriately designed, randomized, double-blind, placebo-controlled clinical trials is just as important for industry as it is for the scientific community. Additionally, he noted, the food industry can develop and market products consistent with nutritional recommendations. Doing so is challenging for industry, he observed, because recommendations such as the DGA revolve around dietary patterns, not necessarily individual products, and consumers must make their own choices from among this panoply of products. He added that the food industry can and does collaborate with government agencies on effective ways to communicate the value of products. Finally, he said, the food industry will continue to partner with industry, scientific, academic, and governmental organizations to inform and educate the public and the medical community about nutrition's vital role in promoting healthy aging.

NUTRIENT GAPS ACROSS THE LIFESPAN AND THE ROLE OF SUPPLEMENTATION IN A HEALTHY DIET[6]

Echoing Morck's message, MacKay began his presentation by emphasizing that "industry is one small piece of this puzzle." Additionally, he stated that, while he recognizes the need to get people to eat more whole grains and vegetables, he also recognizes the dramatic deficiencies in the American diet and practitioners' need for additional tools to help reach nutritional targets. Such targets exist for a reason, he argued. The fact that certain amounts of folic acid or iodine, for example, are important at certain stages of life cannot be ignored, he said. In his opinion, if someone is not getting these nutrients from diet alone, responsible supplementation has a role. He underscored that he works for the dietary supplement industry and represents both the manufacturers of finished products and the ingredient suppliers.

MacKay described several age trends in the 11 shortfall nutrients identified in the 2015-2020 DGA, 10 of which apply across the entire U.S.

[6]This section summarizes information presented by Mr. MacKay.

population aged 2 years and older (vitamin A, vitamin D, vitamin E, vitamin C, folate, choline, calcium, magnesium, fiber, and potassium) and 1 of which applies specifically to premenopausal females (iron). Within these 11 nutrients are 5 of public health concern, he said, nutrients for which underconsumption has been linked to adverse health outcomes: calcium, vitamin D, fiber, potassium, and iron. In adults aged 71 and older, these same shortfalls exist, and in dramatic numbers, MacKay observed. According to the 2015 report of the Dietary Guidelines Advisory Committee (DGAC), 71 percent of men and 81 percent of women have calcium intakes below the Estimated Average Requirement (EAR); 93 percent of men and 97 percent of women have vitamin D levels below the EAR; 96 percent of men and 87 percent of women have fiber levels below the Adequate Intake (AI); and 97 percent of both men and women have potassium levels below the AI.

MacKay reiterated that the consequences of these insufficiencies can be significant. So if efforts to get people to eat better are not working or they are unable to eat vegetables, for example, because they have no teeth, he said, "you need to come up with a solution." He stressed the importance of practitioners understanding their patients' points of reference. If the DASH or Mediterranean diet, for example, is far removed from a patient's point of reference, he said, it is essential to help that person meet those targeted nutrient intakes.

MacKay noted that the numbers in the 2015 DGAC report regarding shortfall nutrients are based on food intake. Biomarker data in the CDC's *Second Nutrition Report* show similar shortfalls in the U.S. population, he observed, with the prevalence of nutrient deficiencies not changing much between 1999 and 2006.

Acknowledging the controversy around the impact of long-chain omega-3 fatty acids, MacKay remarked that the intake of these nutrients among the U.S. population is on par with that of the populations of countries at the lowest levels (i.e., less than or equal to 4 percent of total fatty acids are EPA + DHA) (Stark et al., 2016). Whether one obtains these nutrients by eating anchovies or sardines, as MacKay said he does, or by taking supplements, he argued that there are reasons to consume the levels recommended by the American Heart Association and others.

MacKay remarked that many experts have expressed discomfort with supplements because of concern that people will take them instead of eating well. He noted, however, that based on work by Bailey and colleagues (2013a,b), the top three reasons people take supplements are to improve health, to maintain health, and to supplement the diet. He interprets these results to mean that people who take supplements are not taking them because they do not like vegetables, for example, or because they think that if they take the supplement, they will not have to eat well. Rather, he said, typical supplement users tend to visit their doctor, not smoke, and eat a healthy diet. The real challenge of the industry, in his opinion, is getting the supplements into the hands of the people who need them most.

Evidence on the Population-Level Effects of Dietary Supplements

MacKay went on to describe results, based on NHANES 2003-2006 data, showing that when intakes of dietary supplements were accounted for in addition to food intakes, a smaller percentage of the population fell below the EAR for a number of nutrients (Fulgoni et al., 2011). Fulgoni and colleagues (2011), he explained, estimated nutrient intakes from three different sources: foods with naturally occurring nutrients; all foods, including both those with naturally occurring nutrients and those enriched or fortified; and all foods plus supplements. He showed results for eight of the nutrients examined: vitamin D, vitamin E, folate, vitamin A, calcium, thiamin, vitamin C, and iron (see Figure 5-6). When only foods with naturally occurring nutrients (i.e., excluding fortified foods) were taken into account, the percentages falling below the EAR for these eight nutrients ranged from around 25 percent (iron) to close to 100 percent (vitamin D).

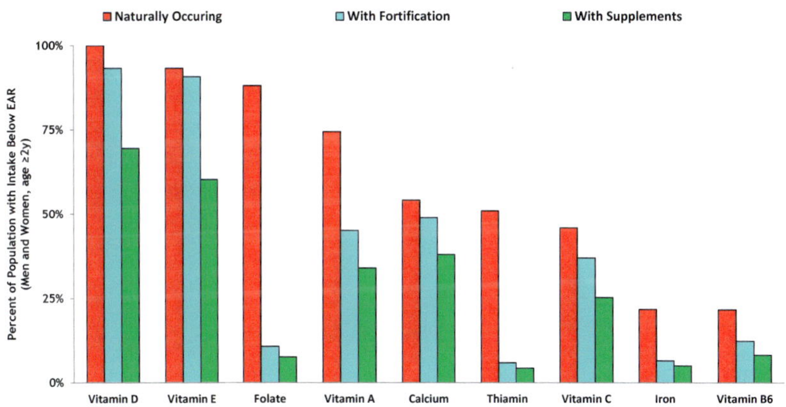

FIGURE 5-6 Percentage of the U.S. population aged 2 years and older with nutrient intakes below Estimated Average Requirements (EARs), taking into account either (1) only intake of foods with naturally occurring nutrients ("naturally occurring"); (2) intake of all foods, including fortified foods ("with fortification"); or (3) intake of all foods plus dietary supplements ("with supplements").
SOURCES: Presented by D. MacKay, September 14, 2016. Adapted with permission of the *Journal of Nutrition*, American Society for Nutrition, from Fulgoni et al., 2011.

When all foods were taken into account, these percentages decreased (i.e., greater percentages of the population met the EARs). And when all foods plus dietary supplements were taken into account, these percentages decreased even further. MacKay reported that the same set of data show that a slightly greater but still very small percentage of supplement users than nonusers were above the Tolerable Upper Intake Level for some nutrients (Bailey et al., 2012).

Women Who Are Pregnant

Women who are pregnant are a highly sensitive subpopulation, MacKay continued, for which three key nutrients are especially important: iron, folic acid, and iodine. There are well-documented consequences of shortfalls of each of these three nutrients, he noted. He explained, however, that the challenges in this regard are tricky because 50 percent of pregnancies are unplanned.

MacKay explained that iron is considered a nutrient of public health concern for women capable of becoming pregnant, with consequences for both the pregnancy and offspring. The folic acid recommendation (i.e., that women capable of becoming pregnant should consume 400 mcg of synthetic folic acid daily from fortified foods and/or supplements) is intended not to meet targeted levels but to provide protection against neural tube defects and is specific to supplemental folic acid. MacKay noted that with respect to iodine, a cluster of concerned physicians, including members of the American Thyroid Association, the Endocrine Society, the Teratology Society, and the American Association of Clinical Endocrinologists, are seeing a subchronic insufficiency of this nutrient in the United States. All of these associations have policy statements recommending that all pregnant U.S. women take a daily prenatal vitamin that contains 150 mcg of iodine in the form of potassium iodide.

Older Adults

In addition to the shortfall nutrients listed above, MacKay identified protein and vitamin B12 as two additional nutrients to consider among older adults. While protein is not a shortfall nutrient, he noted that emerging evidence is beginning to demonstrate benefits of protein intakes above the Recommended Daily Allowance (RDA) levels, especially for older adults and for hospitalized individuals recovering from injury. (See also the summaries of the presentations of Mary Ann Johnson in Chapter 2 and Roger Fielding in Chapter 4 with respect to the controversy concerning protein intake in older adults.) Nor is vitamin B12 a shortfall nutrient, he added, but for older adults with atrophic gastritis whose ability to absorb vitamin

B12 is compromised, the 2010 DGA included a recommendation either to include foods fortified with crystalline B12 or to take a dietary supplement. In MacKay's opinion, even if a person is eating healthfully, supplementation may still be important.

To demonstrate the role of supplements in supporting nutrient adequacy among older adults (age 71 and above), MacKay highlighted calcium and vitamin D. He noted that, based on NHANES 2003-2006 data, calcium intake from foods and beverages did not meet the EAR for older persons, with 71 percent of males and 81 percent of females in this age group having intakes below the EAR. For these analyses, he added, calcium from dietary supplements was also considered. When total intake of foods plus beverages plus dietary supplements containing calcium was considered, the proportion of older adults (age 71 and above) below the EAR improved to 55 percent for men and 49 percent for women (DGAC, 2015). The difference was even more dramatic for vitamin D, MacKay said, with almost none of this older population meeting the EAR with food alone, but about half (both men and women) meeting it with supplements.

The Supplement Industry's Role in Promoting Healthy Aging

In summary, MacKay said, the "lens" of the dietary supplement industry is that, based on the science, significant proportions of the population have inadequate nutrient intakes, and nutrient supplementation is a safe, practical means of improving those intakes. Thus, he explained, the role of the industry in supporting healthy aging is to promote responsible use of dietary supplements in combination with a healthy diet as a way to ensure nutrient adequacy. He noted that the industry takes on this role at both the population and the individual levels.

Industry efforts to promote healthy aging at the population level, MacKay elaborated, include investing in a series of health care cost analyses (i.e., conducting economic analyses to estimate the health care cost savings associated with achieving targeted nutrient intakes for certain disease conditions, such as adequate calcium and vitamin D intakes for bone health); advocating for a multivitamin to be included as a choice in food assistance programs (e.g., SNAP, WIC), given that those in need of food assistance tend to have the greatest nutrient gaps; setting an industry guideline for iodine level in prenatal multivitamins (MacKay mentioned that CRN was currently running a study to evaluate the impact of this guideline); assembling dossiers for health claims or qualified health claims for magnesium (i.e., with respect to blood pressure) and omega-3 fatty acids; and supporting global humanitarian nutrition initiatives, such as Vitamin Angels and Sight and Life.

MacKay explained that industry efforts to promote healthy aging at the individual level (i.e., to meet individual recommendations) revolve around the products. He stated that dietary supplements are science-based products formulated for specific populations (i.e., by life stage and sex). A multivitamin for a woman who is pregnant, for example, is based on one set of nutrient needs, while a multivitamin for a woman who is menstruating is based on another. Additionally, MacKay continued, the industry makes products to complement certain types of diets, such as vegan (e.g., vegan sources of long-chain fatty acids), vegetarian, and lactose-free diets. He noted that the industry also provides products in alternative and creative delivery forms (e.g., powder, liquid, tablet, capsule, gel cap, gummy).

Finally, MacKay addressed managing consumer expectations. "You cannot ignore the push toward sensationalism with aging," he said, as he showed a slide with an image of a television set, with two television personalities in the foreground and on the set in the background the words "The Miracle Pill to Stop Aging." Responsible messaging, he asserted, emphasizes that there is no miracle pill and that people should talk to their physicians. As an example, he mentioned CRN's supplement advertising program, a 10-year program conducted through the Better Business Bureau but with CRN-hired attorneys who challenge supplement manufacturers to either provide substantiation or change the message if substantiation is inadequate.

DISCUSSION WITH THE AUDIENCE

Following MacKay's talk, he and the other speakers in the session participated in an open discussion with the audience. Johanna Dwyer opened the discussion by mentioning the fact sheets on dietary supplements issued by ODS. She commented on problems with the dissolution and disintegration of some supplements and remarked that some of these products may not have the intended effects because they are not absorbed. MacKay responded that this is one of the reasons biomarkers of intake and status are so important in expensive, large studies and need to be collected at baseline and over the course of the study (so it is clear, in the study, whether the product had an effect). Additionally, he noted, monographs of the U.S. Pharmacopeial Convention (USP) include specifications for dissolution. He explained that USP conducts testing to ensure that these products are in compliance with its standards, and while those standards are voluntary, they are mandatory if a company carries the USP seal. To meet USP standards, he continued, a product needs to dissolve based on how dissolution for that product is defined. While this is "not a perfect situation," he said, the industry is aware of the challenge. He stated that when marketing, responsible companies include only claims with evidence (e.g., "twice as absorbable").

An audience member asked what types of research the food industry has been effective in supporting and areas in which, looking ahead, the industry could focus in this regard. Morck replied that what is of great interest to the industry is research results that can be used to support patents or proprietary use of ingredients or processes so that a unique product can be differentiated from its market competitors. Historically, he noted, much of that research has been on bioactive components of a healthy diet (e.g., bioactives such as bioflavonoids or curcumin that are suspected of being associated with a healthy diet). The challenge, he said, is that many research questions are related to disease outcomes (e.g., whether a product affects blood pressure or gastrointestinal conditions or symptoms). He added that a product may in fact improve certain health outcomes, but if these outcomes are associated with improving disease symptoms, the FDA considers the product a drug, not a "food." He explained that there may be areas in which a product consisting of food-derived ingredients may have therapeutic value, and sophisticated tests and tools exist to show that the product may be effective at the physiological or cellular level, but the regulatory paradigm is interpreted "narrowly." Individuals with Alzheimer's disease, for example, are viewed as having the same nutritional requirements as do other individuals in the population. Thus in the current paradigm, Morck said, there is no justification for a medical food for individuals with this condition. He argued that the use of population-based, epidemiological models to set nutrient requirements appropriate for the "general healthy population" fails to consider that patients with disease fall outside this definition. Thus, he believes that new definitions of individual variability in needed nutrient levels are desperately needed to advance this field. He added that in the area of research on infant formula, it took 10 years of evidence showing that specialized hydrolyzed protein formula could be beneficial for babies susceptible to cow's milk allergy before the weight of evidence became compelling enough to obtain a qualified health claim.

MacKay mentioned the Physicians Health Study II again, which showed a reduction in cancer risk associated with multivitamin use, and noted that companies provided multivitamins to 11,000 physicians for 10 years with no expectation regarding outcomes. He described any added effect of a multivitamin in reducing the risk of heart disease, for example, beyond state-of-the-art medical treatment as a "pretty heavy lift," yet companies provided their products for this study at no cost. In fact, he said, the multivitamins did show benefits. Subsequently, he added, CRN conducted a secondary analysis and showed that the effects differed depending on diet. "So the industry is willing to put the money forward," he concluded.

A member of the audience commented on the industry's recognition of the importance of funding research to better understand the population-level effects of components of the diet. For example, General Mills identified whole grains as a focus of research before they became part of the DGA. This research, the audience member noted, has helped build a database that can advance understanding of the relationship between whole grains and health and has impacted how General Mills thinks about its grain products, particularly cereals.

Maha Tahiri, Food Forum member, added that consumer research is another area of research to which the food industry contributes. One of the gaps in the DGA, she observed, is that people do not follow the guidelines. There is much to understand about barriers and motivators, she suggested. Food companies do this type of research, she said, that is, research focused not on branded products but on ethnography. As an example, she noted that General Mills has 15 years of data on what motivates people to lose weight, showing that these motivators are very different for different populations. She told of one researcher who asked a low-income mother who was participating in one of these studies to describe a healthy meal. The woman replied, "pot pie." According to Tahiri, the woman thought that because pot pie has dairy, starch, and vegetables in it, it is healthy. So when the message is to eat more fresh fruits and vegetables, she said, different people interpret that message differently. She believes that through this research, industry can help build a better understanding of what motivates consumers, which in turn can inform efforts to improve the effectiveness of the DGA. "I really see that there is an opportunity for us to share some of our knowledge . . . and what motivates [consumers] and really reaching what we all want, which is for [consumers] to follow the dietary guidelines," Tahiri said.

Dwyer commented on the popular phrase, "70 is the new 50" and asked the panelists whether, therefore, 90 is the new 70. Reuben responded, "Maybe." He identified three factors to consider: (1) how well one takes care of oneself, including exercise; (2) genetics; and (3) luck. In his opinion, luck is often discounted with respect to health. He mentioned having many patients in their 90s who are still working. Most of them, he said, are artists.

A member of the audience commented about the need to temper some of the positive findings regarding progress made by the food industry. For example, the audience member noted, a third-party University of North Carolina evaluation found that the Healthy Weight Commitment Foundation's removal of 6.4 trillion calories from the food supply translates to about 90 fewer calories per person per day. As another example, while calories are declining in the restaurant sector because of mandatory menu labeling that will go into effect in 2017, this commenter believes the restaurant industry has made minimal progress in reducing saturated fat or sodium. In response, Morck called for appropriately validated biomarkers of nutritional status that he suggested should be as easy and convenient to use as a blood pressure cuff. He imagined something that would be on one's phone and could be used to scan a menu in a restaurant to find out exactly what one was eating. "Without knowledge of what we are eating, he said, "we can't make knowledgeable choices."

Finally, a question was raised about the appropriate nutrition for patients who are going through chemotherapy, for example, and what physicians need to do to advocate in this regard in addition to considering the impact of older age and coexisting nutrient deficiencies. The questioner noted that she has watched patients undergo chemotherapy with no nutritional guidance, and that some physicians even tell their patients to stay away from multivitamins. In response, Stoody agreed with others who had urged that everyone has a role in promoting healthy eating and also agreed on the importance of the consumer. Regarding the DGA, she emphasized that the guidelines are about prevention of chronic disease and promotion of healthy eating, but not treatment. In her opinion, the promotion of healthy eating in treatment is a broader conversation that should involve multiple agencies working together.

6

Healthy Aging: What Is It? Are There Acceptable Markers to Utilize in Developing Strategies to Promote It?

Moderator Simin Meydani, director, Jean Mayer U.S. Department of Agriculture (USDA) Human Nutrition Research Center on Aging, Tufts University, opened the final session of the workshop, a panel discussion, with introductory remarks on how the notion of successful, or healthy, aging has changed over time to encompass more than simply the absence of disease or functional impairment. She then asked each of the four panelists of this session to provide their reflections on the workshop presentations and discussions. These comments were followed by an open discussion with the audience.

MEYDANI'S REMARKS

Meydani began by presenting some of her thoughts on healthy aging, informed by the workshop discussion. First, she called attention to some aging statistics that show, she said, "the burden that this could have" on society. One is that in the 1930s, for every retiree, another 16 people were still working, while by 2030, there will be only 2.2 working people per retiree. Another, Meydani said, is the cost associated with the care of chronic diseases. In her opinion, then, developing strategies for increasing the "health span" is critical, both socially and economically. Developing these strategies in turn will require understanding what leads to successful aging, she asserted, including the genetic, lifestyle (including psychosocial interactions), and environmental factors that determine both rate of aging and disease susceptibility. She stated that as yet, there is no consensus on what these factors are—that is, what constitutes healthy aging—a question that remains a major challenge for the field.

Healthy aging used to be defined in terms of the absence of disease, Meydani continued, whereas today's definitions revolve around an understanding that healthy aging is not merely synonymous with lack of disease or functional impairment. She referred to early work by Rowe and Kahn (1987), who, in addition to freedom from disease and disability, considered successful aging to be characterized by having high cognitive and physical functioning, social and productive engagement, and resilience. As one example of the many subsequent attempts to develop an index of successful aging, she cited a study of 2,663 elderly persons (aged 65-100) in the Mediterranean basin. She explained that Tyrovolas and colleagues (2014) found that a multidomain approach—one that accounted for low probability of disease and disability ("clinical characteristics"), high cognitive and physical capacity ("lifestyle characteristics"), and active participation through social activities ("psychosocial-economic characteristics")—better predicted different health outcomes (e.g., use of health care services) than any single domain indicator. She called attention to the fact that in this study, lifestyle characteristics accounted for 48 percent of the variance in successful aging, while psychosocial-economic factors accounted for 23 percent, leaving only 38 percent explained by clinical characteristics.

Meydani also emphasized that studies of successful aging vary considerably in the proportion of individuals considered to have aged successfully depending on how successful aging is defined. She explained that studies of self-rated successful aging result in much higher percentages of successful aging relative to studies based on the definitions of health care workers (Depp and Jeste, 2006). For Meydani, this trend raises an important question: Who should define successful aging, and should older people themselves be providing input?

Meydani referred to other work showing that cognitive performance declines more rapidly with increasing age among people with limited as opposed to average social engagement, and that it declines more slowly among people with more extensive social connections (Haslam et al., 2014). She views social interactions among older adults as important not only for their cognitive functioning but also for the opportunities they provide for food and nutrition interventions (i.e., delivery of healthy foods).

To conclude, Meydani reiterated that there are many ways to define successful aging, including both objectively and subjectively. She observed that while most older people may not meet objective definitions of successful aging, they do meet subjective measures (Jeste et al., 2010). From the perspective of older adults, she asserted, the absence of disease is much less important than independent living, self-rated successful aging, life satisfaction, and several other factors.

PANELIST REMARKS

Following Meydani's presentation, each of the four panelists was asked to present 5 minutes of thoughts on healthy aging.

"Successful aging is living," began Frank Busta, director emeritus, National Center for Food Protection and Defense, and professor emeritus of food biology, University of Minnesota. "Even if you have an illness and disease, you bypass that, and you live." As a microbiologist, he was delighted that the microbiome is being examined over the lifespan, and he suspects that in the near future, this knowledge will have a tremendous influence on healthy aging, given that only part of what people ingest is used to support them directly, with the remainder supporting their microbiome. The many aspects of healthy aging, he continued, including bone structure, skeletal muscle, digestive tract health, appropriate weight, and others, create what he described as a "challenge of choices." In his opinion, the social aspects of healthy aging are extremely important. He observed that he had not heard much about behavior modification at the workshop, yet in his opinion, it is "terribly significant." People know what they should be eating, he asserted, but so many things are associated with food (e.g., socializing, entertainment) that behavioral change is a "tremendous challenge." Some people are capable of meeting this challenge, he suggested, but many have a very difficult time with it, especially those struggling with overweight or obesity. He knows many older people who say, "I am going to enjoy myself. If it cuts 5 years off my life, so be it," an attitude that also raises questions about when in a person's life it is no longer appropriate to intervene.

Mary Ann Johnson observed that much of the workshop discussion had revolved around what she described as "aging process markers." By aging process, she meant the fundamental biological processes of aging. Among gerontologists, whether a process is part of aging or a disease is often the topic of extended conversation. She referred to a December 2015 series of articles in *Science* on this question. In her opinion, physical function (as measured by walking speed, strength, and so on) and living independently (as measured by social engagement) are two markers of the aging process of particular practical significance. Additionally, she noted, while inflammatory markers may not indicate what is wrong, they indicate that something is wrong. Thus, they serve as integrative markers that cut across multiple domains.

In addition to her comments on markers, Johnson called on nutritionists to learn to speak the language of the people who make daily differences in the lives of older adults (e.g., the aging services community, the medical community). "Gait speed," for example, is something professionals in these other communities understand, she said, whereas deficiencies in vitamin D or B12 are not. More generally, she encouraged thinking about how to be partners with and influence the health care system and to find ways, for example, of incorporating nutrition services into care transitions so that older adults are not readmitted to hospitals so quickly.

A workshop message that reverberated for Janet King was the complexity of the aging process. Aging does not begin at age 50, 70, or 90 but in utero, she observed. Because aging is a lifelong process, she continued, healthy aging requires thinking about the lifespan from the very beginning. Moreover, she added, people age differently, some faster than others. When thinking about interventions, she stressed the importance of keeping in mind the socioeconomic context of aging and ensuring that recommendations for interventions can apply to everyone. While speakers at the workshop had identified improving social contacts and cognitive function, for example, as important healthy aging interventions, she works in the poorest part of Oakland, California, where many elderly people lack the resources to participate in those interventions. She suggested identifying key targets that are simple and easy to comprehend and can be communicated to the public. She cited maintaining a certain walking gait (e.g., being able to walk 1 mile in 15 minutes) as an example of something everyone can understand.

Regarding what people should be eating for healthy aging, King found it difficult to offer an answer because no one food can serve this purpose. Despite all the talk about fruits and vegetables, she believes it is time to look critically at nutrient recommendations and start thinking about Dietary Reference Intakes (DRIs) for people aged 51-70 and 71 and older, and then translate those nutrient requirements into food patterns and simple targets. In her opinion, not even ChooseMyPlate is simple enough. She suggested a recommendation such as, "Make sure you have a good source of protein once a day." Not only would meeting that recommendation result in ingesting many micronutrients, but also, according to King, some experts are beginning to think that protein needs may grow higher as one ages and that older adults tend to reduce their protein intakes naturally.

King also observed that this workshop had been a meeting primarily of nutritionists. While nutrition clearly plays a role in the aging process, she asserted, so do many other disciplines as well. In her opinion, it is critical that the issue of healthy aging be addressed in a multidisciplinary way, not through food alone.

The fourth and final panelist, David Reuben, suggested that older people are "painted" as adults with gray hair and wrinkles. "In fact, they are not," he said. He acknowledged many people's desire for 90 to be the new 70. If someone's goal is to be 70 at 90, he suggested, then some of the traditional biomarkers of successful aging are the appropriate focus. However, he argued, it takes a lot of work to be 70 at 90, and many people do not want to work that hard. Moreover, he added, geriatricians work with many frail people, often with incurable diseases such as Alzheimer's.

Rather than geriatricians telling people "this" is how they should be at 90 or at 85, he said, "it's really about what you [the patient] think you should be at 90 or 85 or now through the next 5 years." He commented on the body of literature that exists on the topic of goal setting and goal attainment and suggested that it may be a useful resource. In his practice, he sits down with patients and asks them what they want to achieve. Some of his patients want to be able to watch television with their families, have people over, visit, and so on. He helps them set goals and develop a strategy for meeting those goals, even though sometimes the goals may not resonate with him as a physician.

While Meydani agreed with Reuben that seeking input from older adults about what matters to them is important, she also stressed the need to develop some tangible measures of successful aging. She argued that health care providers need markers to identify at-risk people and know when intervention is appropriate, governments need markers to develop recommendations for older people regarding nutritional intakes or other lifestyle changes, and the food industry needs markers so they can develop products to meet targets.

PANEL DISCUSSION WITH THE AUDIENCE

Following these remarks, Busta asked about public use of the *Dietary Guidelines for Americans* (DGA). Angie Tagtow, Food Forum member, replied that any federal agency that implements a food or nutrition program is supposed to apply the guidelines. Thus, she asserted evaluating the impact of the DGA requires examining all of their federal applications and the number of individuals, families, and communities that are impacted by these federal programs. She noted that the Center for Nutrition Policy and Promotion (CNPP) also relies on practitioners and policy makers to apply the guidelines, which she said is more difficult to measure. She cautioned against making any direct connection between the DGA and overall population health given the numerous confounding variables. She also encouraged looking beyond individual-level interventions and adopting a more systematic approach and, she said, "calling everybody to the table." Meydani asked whether there is a record of how many people have actually visited ChooseMyPlate.gov. Tagtow replied that CNPP measures a wide array of process outputs as part of its Web analytics. To illustrate, she noted that as of the week before the workshop, SuperTracker, an online tool designed to help individuals apply the DGA, had almost 7.4 million registered users. She commented that the small size of the agency is a limiting factor with respect to reaching all 321 million Americans, which in her opinion makes it all the more important that other federal agencies as well as intermediaries apply the guidelines.

Recognizing how difficult the DGA process is, having worked on the guidelines herself in the past, Wendy Johnson-Askew challenged the process. "They [the guidelines] were intended for healthy individuals," she said, "and our population is not healthy." In her opinion, the guidelines need to be translated for individuals based on where they are, not "where we think they should be."

Johnson-Askew also responded to Busta's remarks about behavior. Even in the context of the socioecological model, she said, the individual is still at the center, and thus, individual behavior needs to be driven. She challenged the scientific community, especially researchers who examine behavior, to think about ways of understanding the behavior proclivities of individuals so interventions can be tailored to their needs. Meydani agreed that understanding how behavior can be changed will be helpful for implementing nutrition recommendations. However, she argued, the first step to a behavioral change intervention is understanding what needs to be changed. In terms of successful aging, she asserted, it is unclear what needs to be changed. In her opinion, the parameters of successful aging need to be understood before interventions can be developed. For Johnson-Askew, the first step is to understand how behavior can be changed. She made a call to capitalize on what scientists in other fields have been learning about behavioral phenotyping (e.g., in relation to drug adherence).

Sharon Donovan, workshop participant, said she was struck by the demographics of the aging population. "If we are not doing something," she said, "this country is going to be in for a world of hurt." But she also views the current demographics as an opportunity for research. She has observed a disinvestment of the National Institutes of Health (NIH) in nutrition research over the last 20 years. She cited the lack of nutrition research on the 0 to 24-month age group in particular and said she suspects that the same is true of the elderly. Moreover, she noted, most DRIs have not been reevaluated since they were issued. In her opinion, no one really knows what percentage of the older population is meeting recommended nutrient levels. She asked, "Why do we have a cancer moonshot and we don't have a baby boomer moonshot?" She underscored the current opportunity to enroll a very large cohort (i.e., the baby boomers) in long-term studies that could involve lifestyle interventions, supplements, and other factors. She called for building an evidence base with the appropriate outcomes that are going to have an impact and urged considering interventions beyond those that are behavior-based, given the challenges of adult learning. Johnson agreed that answering many of the questions raised in the workshop will require 10-, 20-, or 30-year studies to see how the aging process plays out.

Meydani agreed on the urgency of understanding the needs of older adults, given the impact not just in the United States but around the world. She observed that most of what is known about the nutritional status of older individuals is based on dietary intake. But, she asserted, dietary intake does not necessarily reflect what is going on in the body. For example, she said, while dietary intake of zinc might not be considered low, in fact 20 to 30 percent of older adults have low serum zinc levels, with potential health consequences. Much remains unknown, she observed, and funding for the necessary research is inadequate. She noted that funding for the National Institute on Aging (NIA) has not increased (although Reuben noted later that the NIA has received increased funding, but that funding has been earmarked for research on Alzheimer's disease).

Johanna Dywer mentioned the many National Academies of Sciences, Engineering, and Medicine reports on aging that have been issued over the past 25 years. More important, she said, she recently received a letter from her long-term care insurance carrier notifying her that her quarterly premiums had increased from $375 to $1,400, and that at least a 15 percent increase would follow in 2017. Many people will not be able to pay these increasing premiums, she observed, and the cost of their care will become public responsibility. "There is a tsunami coming of people over 85, and I'm not sure we can deal with that with the kinds of thing we have been talking about," she said. Reuben agreed that these are major societal issues that keep being kicked down the road. By 2030, he noted, 20 percent of the U.S. population will be aged 65 or older, and he suggested that over the next decade or so, "The hand is going to be forced to make the choices to start addressing these problems in real time." Johnson added that conversations around these issues are beginning to take place, including at the federal, state, and local levels. Much of this discussion, she said, is focused on rebalancing long-term care in a way that keeps people at home and out of nursing homes through home- and community-based services. A big part of these services, she observed, is foods and meals.

CLOSING REMARKS

In closing, Meydani asked the panelists whether there are any markers for healthy aging that could be utilized now and if not, what the next step should be toward compiling a set of such markers. Reuben suggested that there are indeed some existing and some emerging physiological and psychological markers, but there is also a third category—personalized markers based on individuals' perceptions of their own healthy aging. King encouraged thinking about early determinants of inappropriate aging processes, such as inflammation. Johnson agreed with Reuben on the need to identify markers based on what older adults themselves consider to be important, but she suggested that markers also need to be developed based on what programs and payers perceive to be important. Finally, Busta said, "I think the marker of successful aging is being proud of how old you are."

References

Adlerberth, I., and A. E. Wold. 2009. Establishment of the gut microbiota in Western infants. *Acta Paediatrica* 98(2):229-238.

Afilalo, J., S. Kim, and S. O'Brien. 2016. Gait speed and operative mortality in older adults following cardiac surgery. *JAMA Cardiology* 1(3):314-321.

American Academy of Pediatrics. 2012. Section on breastfeeding: Breastfeeding and the use of human milk. *Journal of Pediatrics* 129(3):e827-e841.

Ames, B. N. 2006. Low micronutrient intake may accelerate the degenerative diseases of aging through allocation of scarce micronutrients by triage. *Proceedings of the National Academy of Sciences of the United States of America* 103(47):17589-17594.

Arrain, Y., and T. Masud. 2008. Recent recommendations on bisphosphonate-associated osteonecrosis of the jaw. *Dental Update* 35(4):238-240.

Bailey, R. L., V. L. Fulgoni, III, D. R. Keast, and J. T. Dwyer. 2012. Examination of vitamin intakes among U.S. adults by dietary supplement use. *Journal of the Academy of Nutrition and Dietetics* 112(5):657-663.

Bailey, R. L., J. J. Gahche, P. E. Miller, P. R. Thomas, and J. T. Dwyer. 2013a. Why U. S. adults use dietary supplements. *Journal of the American Medical Association* 173(5):355-361.

Bailey, R. L., J. J. Gahche, P. R. Thomas, and J. T. Dwyer. 2013b. Why U.S. children use dietary supplements. *Pediatric Research* 74(6):737-741.

Barker, D. J., and C. Osmond. 1986. Infant mortality, childhood nutrition, and ischaemic heart disease in England and Wales. *Lancet* 1(8489):1077-1081.

Barker, D. J., J. G. Eriksson, T. Forsén, and C. Osmond. 2002. Fetal origins of adult disease: Strength of effects and biological basis. *International Journal of Epidemiology* 31(6):1235-1239.

Barron, E., J. Lara, M. White, and J. C. Mathers. 2015. Blood-borne biomarkers of mortality risk: Systematic review of cohort studies. *PLOS ONE* 10(6):e0127550.

Bea, J. W., C. A. Thomson, B. C. Wertheim, J. S. Nicholas, K. C. Ernst, C. Hu, R. D. Jackson, J. A. Cauley, C. E. Lewis, B. Caan, D. J. Roe, and Z. Chen. 2015. Risk of mortality according to body mass index and body composition among postmenopausal women. *American Journal of Epidemiology* 182(7):585-596.

Beckett, N. S., R. Peters, A. E. Fletcher, J. A. Staessen, L. Liu, D. Dumitrascu, V. Stoyanovsky, R. L. Antikainen, Y. Nikitin, C. Anderson, A. Belhani, F. Forette, C. Rajkumar, L. Thijs, W. Banya, and C. J. Bulpitt. 2008. Treatment of hypertension in patients 80 years or older. *New England Journal of Medicine* 358(18):1887-1898.

Benetos, A., P. Rossignol, A. Cherbuni, L. Joly, T. Grodzicki, C. Rajkumar, T. E. Strandberg, and M. Petrovic. 2015. Polypharmacy in the aging patient: Management of hypertension in octogenarians. *Journal of the American Medical Association* 314(2):170-180.

Biagi, E., C. Franceschi, S. Rampelli, M. Severgnini, R. Ostan, S. Turroni, C. Consolandi, S. Quercia, M. Scurti, D. Monti, M. Capri, P. Brigidi, and M. Candela. 2016. Gut microbiota and extreme longevity. *Current Biology* 26(11):1480-1485.

Bolland, M. J., A. Avenell, J. A. Baron, A. Grey, G. S. MacLennan, G. D. Gamble, and I. R. Reid. 2010. Effect of calcium supplements on risk of myocardial infarction and cardiovascular events: Meta-analysis. *British Medical Journal* 341:c3691.

Bolland, M. J., A. Grey, A. Avenell, G. D. Gamble, and I. R. Reid. 2011. Calcium supplements with or without vitamin D and risk of cardiovascular events: Reanalysis of the Women's Health Initiative limited access dataset and meta-analysis. *British Medical Journal* 342:d2040.

Brandhorst, S., I. Y. Choi, M. Wei, C. W. Cheng, S. Sedrakyan, G. Navarrete, L. Dubeau, L. P. Yap, R. Park, M. Vinciguerra, S. Di Biase, H. Mirzaei, M. G. Mirisola, P. Childress, L. Ji, S. Groshen, F. Penna, P. Odetti, L. Perin, P. S. Conti, Y. Ikeno, B. K. Kennedy, P. Cohen, T. E. Morgan, T. B. Dorff, and V. D. Longo. 2015. A periodic diet that mimics fasting promotes multi-system regeneration, enhanced cognitive performance, and healthspan. *Cell Metabolism* 22(1):86-99.

Breastcancer.org. 2017. *U.S. breast cancer statistics*. http://www. breastcancer. org/symptoms/understand_bc/statistics (accessed January 13, 2017).

Brown, J. M., and S. L. Hazen. 2014. Metaorganismal nutrient metabolism as a basis of cardiovascular disease. *Current Opinion in Lipidology* 25(1):48-53.

Buford, T. W. 2016. Hypertension and aging. *Ageing Research Reviews* 26:96-111.

Bultman, S. J. 2013. Molecular pathways: Gene-environment interactions regulating dietary fiber induction of proliferation and apoptosis via butyrate for cancer prevention. *Clinical Cancer Research* 20(4):799-803.

Bürkle, A., M. Moreno-Villanueva, J. Bernhard, M. Biasco, G. Zondag, J. H. J. Hoeijmakers, O. Toussaint, B. Grubeck-Loebenstein, E. Mocchegiani, S. Collino, E. S. Gonos, E. Sikora, D. Gradinaru, M. Dollé, M. Salmon, P. Kristensen, H. R. Griffiths, C. Libert, T. Grune, N. Breusing, and A. Simm. 2015. MARK-AGE biomarkers of ageing. *Mechanisms of Ageing and Development* 151:2-12.

Caccamo, A., S. Majumder, A. Richardson, R. Strong, and S. Oddo. 2010. Molecular interplay between mammalian target of rapamycin (mTOR), amyloid-beta, and Tau: Effects on cognitive impairments. *Journal of Biological Chemistry* 285(17):13107-13120.

Carmody, R. N., G. K. Gerber, J. M. Luevano, Jr., D. M. Gatti, L. Somes, K. L. Svenson, and P. J. Turnbaugh. 2015. Diet dominates host genotype in shaping the murine gut microbiota. *Cell Host and Microbe* 17(1):72-84.

CDC (U.S. Centers for Disease Control and Prevention). 2013. State-specific healthy life expectancy at age 65 years—United States, 2007-2009. *Morbidity and Mortality Weekly Report* 62(28):561-566.

CDC. 2015. *Heart disease facts*. https://www.cdc.gov/heartdisease/facts.htm (accessed January 13, 2017).

CDC. 2016. *Stroke*. https://www.cdc.gov/stroke (accessed January 13, 2017).

CDC, Health Resources and Services Administration, Indian Health Service, and National Institutes of Health. 2010. Oral Health. *Healthy People 2010*. Hyattsville, MD: National Center for Health Statistics.

Ceglia, L., S. Niramitmahapanya, M. da Silva Morais, D. A. Rivas, S. S. Harris, H. Bischoff-Ferrari, R. A. Fielding, and B. Dawson-Hughes. 2013. A randomized study on the effect of vitamin D_3 supplementation on skeletal muscle morphology and vitamin D receptor concentration in older women. *Journal of Clinical Endocrinology and Metabolism* 98(12):E1927-E1935.

Cerdá, B., F. A. Tomás-Barberán, and J. C. Espín. 2005. Metabolism of antioxidant and chemopreventive ellagitannins from strawberries, raspberries, walnuts, and oak-aged wine in humans: Identification of biomarkers and individual variability. *Journal of Agricultural and Food Chemistry* 53(2):227-235.

Chapkin, R. S., C. Zhao, I. Ivanov, L. A. Davidson, J. S. Goldsby, J. R. Lupton, R. A. Mathai, M. H. Monaco, D. Rai, W. M. Russell, S. M. Donovan, and E. R. Dougherty. 2010. Noninvasive stool-based detection of infant gastrointestinal development using gene expression profiles from exfoliated epithelial cells. *American Journal of Physiology—Gastrointestinal and Liver Physiology* 298(5):G582-G589.

Checkley, L. A., O. Rho, T. Moore, S. Hursting, and J. DiGiovanni. 2011. Rapamycin is a potent inhibitor of skin tumor promotion by 12-O-tetradecanoylphorbol-13-acetate. *Cancer Prevention Research (Philadelphia, PA)* 4(7):1011-1020.

Chen, M. A. 2016. Multimorbidity in older adults with atrial fibrillation. *Clinics in Geriatric Medicine* 32(2):315-329.

Cheng, F. W., X. Gao, D. C. Mitchell, C. Wood, C. D. Still, D. Rolston, and G. L Jensen. 2016a. Body mass index and all-cause mortality among older adults. *Obesity* 24(10):2232-2239.

Cheng, F. W., X. Gao, D. C. Mitchell, C. Wood, D. D. Rolston, C. D. Still, and G. L. Jensen. 2016b. Metabolic health status and the obesity paradox in older adults. *Journal of Nutrition in Gerontology and Geriatrics* 35(3):161-176.

Chew, E. Y., T. E. Clemons, E. Agrón, E., L. J. Launer, F. Grodstein, and P. S. Bernstein. 2015. Effect of omega-3 fatty acids, lutein/zeaxanthin, or other nutrient supplementation on cognitive function: The AREDS2 randomized clinical trial. *Journal of the American Medical Association* 314(8):791-801.

Chiao, Y. A., and P. S. Rabinovitch. 2015. The aging heart. *Cold Spring Harbor Perspectives in Medicine* 5(9):a025148.

Childers, D. K., and D. B. Allison. 2010. The "obesity paradox": A parsimonious explanation for relations among obesity, mortality rate and aging? *International Journal of Obesity* 34(8):1231-1238.

Cooper, W. N., B. Khulan, S. Owens, C. E. Elks, V. Seidel, A. M. Prentice, G. Belteki, K. K. Ong, N. A. Affara, M. Constância, and D. B. Dunger. 2012. DNA methylation profiling at imprinted loci after periconceptional micronutrient supplementation in humans: Results of a pilot randomized controlled trial. *FASEB Journal* 26(5):1782-1790.

Dabelea, D., E. J. Mayer-Davis, S. Saydah, G. Imperatore, B. Linder, J. Divers, R. Bell, A. Badaru, J. W. Talton, T. Crume, A. D. Liese, A. T. Merchant, J. M. Lawrence, K. Reynolds, L. Dolan, L. L. Liu, and R. F. Hamman. 2014. Prevalence of type 1 and type 2 diabetes among children and adolescents from 2001 to 2009. *Journal of the American Medical Association* 311(17):1778-1786.

Dam, T. T., K. W. Peters, M. Fragala, P. M Cawthon, T. B. Harris, R. McLean, M. Shardell, D. E. Alley, A. Kenny, L. Ferrucci, J. Guralnik, D. P. Kiel, S. Kritchevsky, M. T. Vassileva, and S. Studenski. 2014. An evidence-based comparison of operational criteria for the presence of sarcopenia. *Journal of Gerontology* 69(5):584-590.

Dato, S., D. Bellizzi, G. Rose, and G. Passarino. 2016. The impact of nutrients on the aging rate: A complex interaction of demographic, environmental and genetic factors. *Mechanisms of Ageing and Development* 154:49-61.

David, L. A., C. F. Maurice, R. N. Carmody, D. B. Gootenberg, J. E. Button, B. E. Wolfe, A. V. Ling, A. S. Devlin, Y. Varma, M. A. Fischbach, S. B. Biddinger, R. J. Dutton, and P. J. Turnbaugh. 2014. Diet rapidly and reproducibly alters the human gut microbiome. *Nature* 505(7484):559-563.

Davidson, L. A., Y. H. Jiang, J. R. Lupton, and R. S. Chapkin. 1995. Noninvasive detection of putative biomarkers for colon cancer using fecal messenger RNA. *Cancer Epidemiology, Biomarkers & Prevention* 4(6):643-647.

de Cabo, R., D. Carmona-Gutierrez, M. Bernier, M. N. Hall, and F. Madeo. 2014. The search for antiaging interventions: From elixirs to fasting regimens. *Cell* 157(7):1515-1526.

Depp, C. A., and D. V. Jeste. 2006. Definitions and predictors of successful aging: A comprehensive review of larger quantitative studies. *American Journal of Geriatric Psychiatry* 14(1):6-20.

DGAC (Dietary Guidelines Advisory Committee). 2015. *Scientific report of the 2015 Dietary Guidelines Advisory Committee*. Washington, DC: HHS and USDA.

Dickinson, M. H., C. T. Farley, R. J. Full, M. A. Koehl, R. Kram, and S. Lehman. 2000. How animals move: An integrative review. *Science* 288(5463):100-106.

Dominguez-Bello, M. G., M. J. Blaser, R. E. Ley, and R. Knight. 2011. Development of the human gastrointestinal microbiota and insights from high-throughput sequencing. *Gastroenterology* 140(6):1713-1719.

Dominguez-Salas, P., S. E. Moore, D. Cole, K. A. da Costa, S. E. Cox, R. A. Dyer, A. J. Fulford, S. M. Innis, R. A. Waterland, S. H. Zeisel, A. M. Prentice, and B. J. Hennig. 2013. DNA methylation potential: Dietary intake and blood concentrations of one-carbon metabolites and cofactors in rural African women. *American Journal of Clinical Nutrition* 97(6):1217-1227.

Dominguez-Salas, P., S. E. Moore, M. S. Baker, A. W. Bergen, S. E. Cox, R. A. Dyer, A. J. Fulford, Y. Guan, E. Laritsky, M. J. Silver, G. E. Swan, S. H. Zeisel, S. M. Innis, R. A. Waterland, A. M. Prentice, and B. J. Hennig. 2014. Maternal nutrition at conception modulates DNA methylation of human metastable epialleles. *Nature Communications* 5:3746.

Dutton, R. J., and P. J. Turnbaugh. 2012. Taking a metagenomic view of human nutrition. *Current Opinion in Clinical Nutrition and Metabolic Care* 15(5):448-454.

Estruch, R., E. Ros, J. Salas-Salvadó, M. I. Covas, D. Corella, F. Arós, E. Gómez-Gracia, V. Ruiz-Gutiérrez, M. Fiol, J. Lapetra, R. M. Lamuela-Raventos, L. Serra-Majem, X. Pintó, J. Basora, M. A. Muñoz, J. V. Sorlí, J. A. Martínez, and M. A. Martínez-González. 2013. Primary prevention of cardiovascular disease with a Mediterranean diet. *New England Journal of Medicine* 368(14):1279-1290.

Ettehad, D., C. Emdin, A. Kiran, S. Anderson, T. Callender, J. Emberson, J. Chalmers, A. Rodgers, and K. Rahimi. 2016. Blood pressure lowering for prevention of cardiovascular disease and death: A systematic review and meta-analysis. *Lancet* 387(10022):957-967.

Everitt, A. V., C. D. Shorey, and M. A. Ficarra. 1985. Skeletal muscle aging in the hind limb of the old male Wistar rat: Inhibitory effect of hypophysectomy and food restriction. *Archives of Gerontology and Geriatrics* 4(2):101-115.

Federal Interagency Forum on Aging-related Statistics. 2016. *Older Americans 2016: Key indicators of well-being*. https://agingstats.gov/docs/LatestReport/OA2016.pdf (accessed January 18, 2017).

Ferrucci, L., and S. Studenski. 2011. Clinical problems of aging. In *Harrison's Principles of Internal Medicine*, 18th ed., edited by D. L. Longo, A. S. Fauci, D. L. Kasper, S. L. Hauser, J. L. Jameson, and J. Loscalzo. New York: McGraw Hill. Pp. 570-587.

Ferrucci, L., T. B. Harris, J. M. Guralnik, R. P. Tracy, M. C. Corti, H. J. Cohen, B. Penninx, M. Pahor, R. Wallace, and R. J. Havlik. 1999. Serum IL-6 level and the development of disability in older persons. *Journal of the American Geriatrics Society* 47(6):639-646.

Fleg, J. 1986 Alterations in cardiovascular structure and function with advancing age. *American Journal of Cardiology* 57(5):C33-C44.

Flegal, K. M., B. K. Kit, H. Orpana, and B. I. Graubard. 2013. Association of all-cause mortality with overweight and obesity using standard body mass index categories: A systematic review and meta-analysis. *Journal of the American Medical Association* 309(1):71-82.

Freedman, D. S., W. H. Dietz, R. Tang, G. A. Mensah, M. G. Bond, E. M. Urbina, S. Srinivasan, and G. S. Berenson. 2004. The relation of obesity throughout life to carotid intima-media thickness in adulthood: The Bogalusa Heart Study. *International Journal of Obesity and Related Metabolic Disorders* 28(1):159-166.

Freedman, D. S., Z. Mei, S. R. Srinivasan, G. S. Berenson, and W. H. Dietz. 2007. Cardiovascular risk factors and excess adiposity among overweight children and adolescents: The Bogalusa Heart Study. *Journal of Pediatrics* 150(1):12-17.

Froman, D. E., A. Ahmed, and J. L. Fieg. 2013. Heart failure in very old adults. *Current Heart Failure Reports* 10(4):387-400.

Fulgoni, III, V. L., D. R. Keast, R. L. Bailey, and J. Dwyer. 2011. Foods, forticants, and supplements: Where do Americans get their nutrients? *Journal of Nutrition* 141(10):1847-1854.

Gaillard, R. 2015. Maternal obesity during pregnancy and cardiovascular development and disease in the offspring. *European Journal of Epidemiology* 30(11):1141-1152.

Halagappa, V. K., Z. Guo, M. Pearson, Y. Matsuoka, R. G. Cutler, F. M. Laferia, and M. P. Mattson. 2007. Intermittent fasting and caloric restriction amelioriate age-related behavioral deficits in the triple-transgenic mouse model of Alzheimer's disease. *Neurobiology of Disease* 26(1):212-220.

Hamman, R. F., R. A. Bell, D. Dabelea, R. B. D'Agostino, Jr., L. Dolan, G. Imperatore, J. M. Lawrence, B. Linder, S. M. Marcovina, E. J. Mayer-Davis, C. Pihoker, B. L. Rodriguez, and S. Saydah. 2014. The SEARCH for Diabetes in Youth study: Rationale, findings, and future directions. *Diabetes Care* 37(12):3336-3344.

Hansen, M. A., K. Overgaard, B. J. Riis, and C. Christiansen. 1991. Role of peak bone mass and bone loss in postmenopausal osteoporosis: 12-year study. *British Medical Journal* 303(6808):961-964.

Hardy, S. E., Y. Kang, S. A. Studenski, and H. B. Degenholtz. 2011. Ability to walk 1/4 mile predicts subsequent disability, mortality, and health care costs. *Journal of General Internal Medicine* 26(2):130-135.

Harrison, D. E., R. Strong, Z. D. Sharp, J. F. Nelson, C. M. Astle, K. Flurkey, N. L. Nadon, J. E. Wilkinson, K. Frenkel, C. S. Carter, M. Pahor, M. A. Javors, E. Fernandez, and R. A. Miller. 2009. Rapamycin fed late in life extends lifespan in genetically heterogeneous mice. *Nature* 1460(7253):392-395.

Harrison, D. E., R. Strong, D. B. Allison, B. N. Ames, C. M. Astle, H. Atamna, E. Fernandez, K. Flurkey, M. A. Javors, N. L. Nadon, J. F. Nelson, S. Pletcher, J. W. Simpkins, D. Smith, J. E. Wilkinson, and R. A. Miller. 2014. Acarbose, 17-α-estradiol, and nordihydroguaiaretic acid extend mouse lifespan preferentially in males. *Aging Cell* 13(2):273-282.

Harvey, A., A. C. Montezano, and R. M. Touyz. 2015. Vascular biology of ageing 0—Implications in hypertension. *Journal of Molecular and Cellular Cardiology* 83:112-121.

Haslam, C., T. Cruwys, and S. A. Haslam. 2014. "The we's have it": Evidence for the distinctive benefits of group engagement in enhancing cognitive health in aging. *Social & Medicine* 120:57-66.

Hattori, M., and T. D. Taylor. 2009. The human intestinal microbiome: A new frontier of human biology. *DNA Research* 16(1):1-12.

Heaney, R. P., S. Abrams, B. Dawson-Hughes, A. Looker, R. Marcus, V. Matkovic, and C. Weaver. 2000. Peak bone mass. *Osteoporosis International* 11(12):985-1009.

HHS (U.S. Department of Health and Human Services) and USDA (U.S. Department of Agriculture). 2015. *Dietary Guidelines for Americans 2015-2020*. https://health.gov/dietaryguidelines/2015/guidelines (accessed January 18, 2017).

Hoffman, H. J., S. Rawal, C. M. Li, and V. B. Duffy. 2016. New chemosensory component in the U.S. National Health and Nutrition Examination Survey (NHANES): First-year results for measured olfactory dysfunction. *Reviews in Endocrine and Metabolic Disorders* 17(2):221-240.

Houston, D. K., B. J. Nicklas, J. Ding, T. B. Harris, F. A. Tylavsky, A. B. Newman, J. S. Lee, N. R. Sahyoun, M. Visser, and S. B. Kritchevsky. 2008. Dietary protein intake is associated with lean mass change in older, community-dwelling adults: The Health, Aging, and Body Composition (Health ABC) Study. *American Journal of Clinical Nutrition* 87(1):150-155.

Hsia, J., G. Heiss, H. Ren, M. Allison, N. C. Dolan, P. Greenland, S. R. Heckbert, K. C. Johnson, J. E. Manson, S. Sidney, and M. Trevisan. 2007. Calcium/vitamin D supplementation and cardiovascular events. *Circulation* 115(7):846-854.

Hughes, V. 2013. The big fat truth. *Nature* 497(7450):428-430.

Inagaki, K., Y. Kurosu, T. Kamiya, F. Kondo, N. Yoshinari, T. Noguchi, E. A. Krall, and R. I. Garcia. 2001. Low metacarpal bone density, tooth loss, and periodontal disease in Japanese women. *Journal of Dental Research* 80(9):1818-1822.

IOM (Institute of Medicine). 2004. *Infant formula: Evaluating the safety of new ingredients*. Washington, DC: The National Academies Press.

IOM. 2011. *Dietary Reference Intakes for calcium and vitamin D*. Washington, DC: The National Academies Press.

Isaacs, B. 1979. Should we treat hypertension in the elderly? *Age and Ageing* 8(2):115-120.

Jang, S., J. Sun, P. Chen, S. Lakshman, A. Molokin, J. M. Harnly, B. T. Vinyard, J. F. Urban, Jr., C. D. Davis, and G. Solano-Aguilar. 2016. Flavanol-enriched cocoa powder alters the intestinal microbiota, tissue and fluid metabolite profiles, and intestinal gene expression in pigs. *Journal of Nutrition* 146(4):673-680.

Jeste, D. V., C. A. Depp, and I. V. Vahia. 2010. Successful cognitive and emotional aging. *World Psychiatry* 9(2):78-84.

Juonala, M., C. G. Magnuseen, G. S. Berenson, A. Venn, T. L. Burns, M. A. Sabin, S. R. Srinivasan, S. R. Daniels, P. H. Davis, W. Chen, C. Sun, M. Cheung, J. S. Viikari, T. Dwyer, and O. T. Raitakari. 2011. Childhood adiposity, adult adiposity, and cardiovascular risk factors. *New England Journal of Medicine* 365(20):1876-1885.

Kamer, A. R., E. Pirraglia, W. Tsui, H. Rusinek, S. Vallabhajosula, L. Mosconi, L. Yi, P. McHugh, R. G. Craig, S. Svetcov, R. Linker, C. Shi, L. Glodzik, S. Williams, P. Corby, D. Saxena, and M. J. de Leon. 2015. Periodontal disease associates with higher brain amyloid load in normal elderly. *Neurobiology of Aging* 36(2):627-633.

Kanis, J. A., D. Hans, C. Cooper, S. Baim, J. P. Bilezikian, N. Binkley, J. A. Cauley, J. E. Compston, B. Dawson-Hughes, G. El-Hajj Fuleihan, H. Johansson, W. D. Leslie, E. M. Lewiecki, M. Luckey, A. Oden, S. E. Papapoulos, C. Poiana, R. Rizzoli, D. A. Wahl, and E. V. McCloskey. 2011. Interpretation and use of FRAX in clinical practice. *Osteoporosis International* 22(9):2395-2411.

Keenan, M. J., M. L. Marco, D. K. Ingram, and R. J. Martin. 2015. Improving healthspan via changes in gut microbiota and fermentation. *Age* 37(5):98.

Keller, K. M., and S. E. Howlett. 2016. Sex differences in the biology and pathology of the aging heart. *Canadian Journal of Cardiology* 32(9):1065-1073.

Kern, J., S. Kern, K. Blennow, H. Zetterberg, M. Waern, X. Guo, A. Börjesson-Hanson, I. Skoog, and S. Östling. 2016. Calcium supplementation and risk of dementia in women with cerebrovascular disease. *Neurology* 87(16):1674-1680.

Kertzer, D. I., and P. Laslett, eds. 1995. *Aging in the past: Demography, society, and old age.* Berkeley, CA: University of California Press.

Klein, S., L. Fontana, V. L. Young, A. R. Coggan, C. Kilo, B. W. Patterson, and B. S. Mohammed. 2004. Absence of an effect of liposuction on insulin action and risk factors for coronary heart disease. *New England Journal of Medicine* 350(25):2549-2557.

Knight, J. M., L. A. Davidson, D. Herman, C. R. Martin, J. S. Goldsby, I. V. Ivanov, S. M. Donovan, and R. S. Chapkin. 2014. Non-invasive analysis of intestinal development in preterm and full term infants using RNA-SEQ: A pilot study. *Nature Scientific Reports* 4:5453.

Kostic, A. D., M. R. Howitt, and W. S. Garrett. 2013. Exploring host-microbiota interactions in animal models and humans. *Genes and Development* 27(7):701-718.

Krall, E. A., B. Dawson-Hughes, A. S. Papas, and R. Garcia. 1994. Tooth loss and skeletal bone density in healthy postmenopausal women. *Osteoporosis International* 4(2):104-109.

Lakatta, E. G. 2015. So! What's aging? Is cardiovascular aging a disease? *Journal of Molecular and Cellular Cardiology* 83:1-13.

Lara, J., E. H. Evans, N. O'Brien, P. J. Moynihan, T. D. Meyer, A. J. Adamson, L. Errington, F. F. Sniehotta, M. White, and J. C. Mathers. 2014. Association of behaviour change techniques with effectiveness of dietary interventions among adults of retirement age: A systematic review and meta-analysis of randomized controlled trials. *BMC Medicine* 12:177.

Lara, J., R. Cooper, J. Nissan, A. T. Ginty, K.-T. Khaw, I. J. Deary, J. M. Lord, D. Kuh, and J. C. Mathers. 2015. A proposed panel of biomarkers of healthy aging. *BMC Medicine* 13:222.

Lee, J. S., J. G. Fischer, and M. A. Johnson. 2010. Food insecurity, food and nutrition programs, and aging: Experiences from Georgia. *Journal of Nutrition for the Elderly* 29(2):116-149.

Li, S., W. Chen, S. R. Srinivasan, M. G. Bond, R. Tang, E. M. Urbina, and G. S. Berenson. 2003. Childhood cardiovascular risk factors and carotid vascular changes in adulthood: The Bogalusa Heart Study. *Journal of the American Medical Association* 290(17):2271-2276.

Macpherson, H., A. Pipingas, and M. P. Pase. 2013. Multivitamin-multimineral supplementation and mortality: A meta-analysis of randomized controlled trials. *American Journal of Clinical Nutrition* 97(2):437-444.

Mannick, J. B., G. Del Guidice, M. Lattanzi, N. M. Valiante, J. Praestgaard, B. Huang, M. A. Lonetto, H. T. Maecker, J. Kovarik, S. Carson, D. J. Glass, and L. B. Klickstein. 2014. mTOR inhibition improves immune function in the elderly. *Science Translational Medicine* 6(268):268ra179.

Martens, E. 2016. Microbiome: Fibre for the future. *Nature* 529(7585):158-159.

Martínez-Lapiscina, E. H., P. Clavero, E. Toledo, R. Estruch, J. Salas-Salvadó, B. San Julián, A. Sanchez-Tainta, E. Ros, C. Valls-Pedret, and M. Á. Martinez-Gonzalez. 2013. Mediterranean diet improves cognition: The PREDIMED-NAVARRA randomised trial. *Journal of Neurology, Neurosurgery & Psychiatry* 84(12):1318-1325.

Matsumoto, M., S. Kurihara, R. Kibe, H. Ashida, and Y. Benno. 2011. Longevity in mice is promoted by probiotic-induced suppression of colonic senescence dependent on upregulation of gut bacterial polyamine production. *PLOS ONE* 6(8):e23652.

Miller, M. S., P. Lekkas, J. M. Braddock, G. P. Farman, B. A. Baliff, T. C. Irving, D. W. Maughan, and J. O. Vigoreaux. 2008. Aging enhances indirect flight muscle fiber performance yet decreases flight ability in Drosophila. *Biophysical Journal* 95(5):2391-2401.

Miller, R. A., D. E. Harrison, C. M. Astle, E. Fernandez, K. Flurkey, M. Han, M. A. Javors, X. Li, N. L. Nadon, J. F. Nelson, S. Pletcher, A. B. Salmon, Z. D. Sharp, S. Van Roekel, L. Winkleman, and R. Strong. 2014. Rapamycin-mediated lifespan increase in mice is dose and sex dependent and metabolically distinct from dietary restriction. *Aging Cell* 13(3):468-477.

Mitchell, S. J., J. Madrigal-Matute, M. Scheibye-Knudsen, E. Fang, M. Aon, J. A. González-Reyes, S. Cortassa, S. Kaushik, M. Gonzalez-Freire, B. Patel, D. Wahl, A. Ali, M. Calvo-Rubio, M. I. Burón, V. Guiterrez, T. M. Ward, H. H. Palacios, H. Cai, D. W. Frederick, C. Hine, F. Broeskamp, L. Habering, J. Dawson, T. M. Beasley, J. Wan, Y. Ikeno, G. Hubbard, K. G. Becker, Y. Zhang, V. A. Bohr, D. L. Longo, P. Navas, L. Ferrucci, D. A. Sinclair, P. Cohen, J. M. Egan, J. R. Mitchell, J. A. Baur, D. B. Allison, R. M. Anson, J. M. Villalba, F. Madeo, A. M. Cuervo, K. J. Pearson, D. K. Ingram, M. Bernier, and R. de Cabo. 2016. Effects of sex, strain, and energy intake on hallmarks of aging in mice. *Cell Metabolism* 23(6):1093-1112.

Moore, A. Z., G. Caturegli, E. J. Metter, S. Makrogiannis, S. M. Resnick, T. B. Harris, and L. Ferrucci. 2014. Difference in muscle quality over the adult life span and biological correlates in the Baltimore Longitudinal Study of Aging. *Journal of the American Geriatrics Society* 62(2):230-236.

Morley, J. E., R. N. Baumgartner, R. Roubenoff, J. Mayer, and K. S. Nair. 2001. Sarcopenia. *Journal of Laboratory and Clinical Medicine* 137(4):231-243.

Morris, M. C., C. C. Tangney, Y. Wang, F. M. Sacks, L. L. Barnes, D. A. Bennett, and N. T. Aggarwal. 2015. MIND diet slows cognitive decline with aging. *Alzheimer's & Dementia* 11(9):1015-1022.

Mozaffarian, D., P. W. Wilson, and W. B. Kannel. 2008. Beyond established and novel risk factors: Lifestyle risk factors for cardiovascular disease. *Circulation* 117(23):3031-3038.

Mozaffarian, D., E. J. Benjamin, A. S. Go, D. K. Arnett, M. J. Blaha, M. Cushman, S. R. Das, S. de Ferranti, J. P. Després, H. J. Fullerton, V. J. Howard, M. D. Huffman, C. R. Isasi, M. C. Jiménez, S. E. Judd, B. M. Kissela, J. H. Lichtman, L. D. Lisabeth, S. Liu, R. H. Mackey, D. J. Magid, D. K. McGuire, E. R. Mohler, III, C. S. Moy, P. Muntner, M. E. Mussolino, K. Nasir, R. W. Neumar, G. Nichol, L. Palaniappan, D. K. Pandey, M. J. Reeves, C. J. Rodriguez, W. Rosamond, P. D. Sorlie, J. Stein, A. Towfighi, T. N. Turan, S. S. Virani, D. Woo, R. W. Yeh, and M. B. Turner. 2016. Heart disease and stroke statistics—2016 update: A report from the American Heart Association. *Circulation* 133(4):e38-e360.

Murphy, R. A., I. Reinders, M. E. Garcia, G. Eiriksdottir, L. J. Launer, R. Benediktsson, V. Gudnason, P. V. Jonsson, and T. B. Harris. 2014. Adipose tissue, muscle, and function: Potential mediators of associations between body weight and mortality in older adults with type 2 diabetes. *Diabetes Care* 37(12):3213-3219.

Murray, C. J., C. Atkinson, K. Bhalia, G. Birbeck, R. Burstein, et al. 2013. The state of U.S. health, 1990-2010: Burden of diseases, injuries, and risk factors. *Journal of the American Medical Association* 310(6):591-608.

Mursu, J., K. Robien, L. J. Harnack, K. Park, and D. R. Jacobs, Jr. 2011. Dietary supplements and mortality rate in older women: The Iowa Women's Health Study. *Archives of Internal Medicine* 171(18):1625-1633.

Nathan, B. M., and A. Moran 2008. Metabolic complications of obesity in childhood and adolescence: More than just diabetes. *Current Opinion Endocrinology, Diabetes, and Obesity* 15(1):21-29.

National Osteoporosis Foundation. 2017. *General facts.* https://www.nof.org/preventing-fractures/general-facts (accessed February 15, 2017).

Nicklas, T. A., S. P. von Duvillard, and G. S. Berenson. 2002. Tracking of serum lipids and lipoproteins from childhood to dyslipidemia in adults: The Bogalusa Heart Study. *International Journal of Sports Medicine* 23(Suppl. 1):S39-S43.

Ning, H., D. R. Labarthe, C. M. Shay, S. R. Daniels, L. Hou, L. Van Horn, and D. M. Lloyd-Jones. 2015. Status of cardiovascular health in U.S. children up to 11 years of age: The National Health and Nutrition Examination Surveys 2003-2010. *Circulation. Cardiovascular Quality and Outcomes* 8(2):164-171.

Office of the Surgeon General. 2004. *Bone health and osteoporosis: A report of the Surgeon General. The burden of bone disease*. Rockville, MD: Office of the Surgeon General. https://www.ncbi.nlm.nih.gov/books/NBK45502 (accessed February 24, 2017).

Oreopoulos, A., K. Kalantar-Zadeh, A. M. Sharma, and G. C. Fonarow. 2009. The obesity paradox in the elderly: Potential mechanisms and clinical implications. *Clinics in Geriatric Medicine* 25(4):643-659.

O'Rourke, M. F., M. E. Safar, and V. Dzau. 2010. The cardiovascular continuum extended: Aging effects on the aorta and microvasculature. *Vascular Medicine* 15(6):461-468.

Pepine, C. J. 1998. The effects of angiotensin-converting enzyme inhibition on endothelial dysfunction: Potential role in myocardial ischemia. *American Journal of Cardiology* 82(10A):23S-27S.

Population Division of the Department of Economic and Social Affairs of the United Nations Secretariat. 2005. *World population prospects. The 2004 revision*. New York: United Nations. http://www.un.org/esa/population/publications/WPP2004/2004Highlights_final revised.pdf (accessed January 18, 2017).

Potten, C. S., R. Schofield, and L. G. Lajtha. 1979. A comparison of cell replacement in bone marrow, testis and three regions of surface epithelium. *Biochimica et Biophysica Acta* 560(2):281-299.

Prentice, R. L., M. B. Pettinger, R. D. Jackson, J. Wactawski-Wende, A. Z. Lacroix, G. L. Anderson, R. T. Chlebowski, J. E. Manson, L. Van Horn, M. Z. Vitolins, M. Datta, E. S. LeBlanc, J. A. Cauley, and J. E. Rossouw. 2013. Health risks and benefits from calcium and vitamin D supplementation: Women's Health Initiative Clinical Trial and Cohort Study. *Osteoporosis International* 24(2):567-580.

Raitakari, O. T., M. Juonala, M. Kähönen, L. Taittonen, T. Laitinen, N. Mäki-Torkko, M. J. Järvisalo, M. Uhari, E. Jokinen, T. Rönnemaa, H. K. Akerblom, and J. S. Viikari. 2003. Cardiovascular risk factors in childhood and carotid artery intima-media thickness in adulthood: The Cardiovascular Risk in Young Finns Study. *Journal of the American Medical Association* 290(17):2277-2283.

Rautava, S., M. C. Collado, S. Salminen, and E. Isolauri. 2012. Probiotics modulate host-microbe interaction in the placenta and fetal gut: A randomized, double-blind, placebo-controlled trial. *Neonatology* 102(3):178-184.

Rawson, N. E., and A. S. LaMantia. 2007. A speculative essay on retinoic acid regulation of neural stem cells in the developing and aging olfactory system. *Experimental Gerontology* 42(1-2):46-53.

Rawson, N. E., G. Gomez, B. J. Cowart, A. Kriete, E. Pribitkin, and D. Restrepo. 2012. Age-associated loss of selectivity in human olfactory sensory neurons. *Neurobiology of Aging* 33(9):1913-1919.

Richards, J. L., Y. A. Yap, K. H. McLeod, C. R. Mackay, and E. Mariño. 2016. Dietary metabolites and the gut microbiota: An alternative approach to control inflammatory and autoimmune diseases. *Clinical and Translational Immunology* 5(5):e82.

Robinson, S., and C. Fall. 2012. Infant nutrition and later health: A review of current evidence. *Nutrients* 4(8):859-874.

Rossouw, J. E., G. L. Anderson, R. L. Prentice, A. Z. LaCroix, C. Kooperberg, M. L. Stefanick, R. D. Jackson, S. A. Beresford, B. V. Howard, K. C. Johnson, J. M. Kotchen, and J. Ockene. 2002. Risks and benefits of estrogen plus progestin in healthy postmenopausal women: Principal results from the Women's Health Initiative randomized controlled trial. *Journal of the American Medical Association* 288(3):321-333.

Rowe, J. W., and R. L. Kahn. 1987. Human aging: Usual and successful. *Science* 237(4811): 143-149.

Russell, R. G., N. B. Watts, F. H. Ebetino, and M. J. Rogers. 2008. Mechanisms of action of bisphosphonates: Similarities and differences and their potential influence on clinical efficacy. *Osteoporosis International* 19(6):733-759.

Sanders, J. L., R. L. Minster, M. M. Barmada, A. M. Matteini, R. M. Boudreau, K. Christensen, R. Mayeux, I. B. Borecki, Q. Zhang, T. Perls, and A. B. Newman. 2014. Heritability of and mortality prediction with a longevity phenotype: The healthy aging index. *Journals of Gerontology Series A: Biological Sciences and Medical Sciences* 69(4):479-485.

Schwartz, S., I. Friedberg, I. Ivanov, L. A. Davidson, J. S. Goldsby, D. B. Dahl, D. Herman, M. Wang, S. M. Donovan, and R. S. Chapkin. 2012. A metagenomic study of diet-dependent interaction between gut micriobiota and host in infants reveals differences in developmental and immune responses. *Genome Biology* 13(4):R32.

Schwingshackl, L., and G. Hoffmann. 2014. Adherence to Mediterranean diet and risk of cancer: A systematic review and meta-analysis of observational studies. *International Journal of Cancer* 135(8):1884-1897.

Siervo, M., J. Lara, S. Chowdhury, A. Ashor, C. Oggioni, and J. C. Mathers. 2015. Effects of the Dietary Approach to Stop Hypertension (DASH) diet on cardiovascular risk factors: A systematic review and meta-analysis. *British Journal of Nutrition* 113(1):1-15.

Sinding, C., L. Puschmann, and T. Hummel. 2014. Is the age-related loss in olfactory sensitivity similar for light and heavy molecules? *Chemical Senses* 39(5):383-390.

Smith, P. J., J. A. Blumenthal, M. A. Babyak, L. Craighead, K. A. Welsh-Bohmer, J. N. Browndyke, T. A. Strauman, and A. Sherwood. 2010. Effects of the dietary approaches to stop hypertension diet, exercise, and 16 caloric restriction on neurocognition in overweight adults with high blood pressure. *Hypertension* 55(6):1331-1338.

Smulyan, H., S. Mookherjee, and M. E. Safar. 2016. The two faces of hypertension: Role of aortic stiffness. *Journal of the American Society of Hypertension* 10(2):175-183.

Sofi, F., F. Cesari, R. Abbate, G. F. Gensini, and A. Casini. 2008. Adherence to Mediterranean diet and health status: Meta-analysis. *British Medical Journal* 337:a1344.

Sonnenburg, E. D., S. A. Smits, M. Tikhonov, S. K. Higginbottom, N. S. Wingreen, and J. L. Sonnenburg. 2016. Diet-induced extinctions in the gut microbiota compound over generations. *Nature* 529(7585):212-215.

Sonnenburg, J. L., and F. Bäckhed. 2016. Diet-microbiota interactions as moderators of human metabolism. *Nature* 535(7610):56-64.

SPRINT (Systolic Blood Pressure Intervention Trial) Research Group, J. T. Wright, Jr., J. D. Williamson, P. K. Whelton, J. K. Snyder, K. M. Sink, M. V. Rocco, D. M. Reboussin, M. Rahman, S. Oparil, C. E. Lewis, P. L. Kimmel, K. C. Johnson, D. C. Goff, Jr., L. J. Fine, J. A. Cutler, W. C. Cushman, A. K. Cheung, and W. T. Ambrosius. 2015. A randomized trial of intensive versus standard blood-pressure control. *New England Journal of Medicine* 373(22):2103-2116.

Stark, K. D., M. E. Van Elswyk, H. R. Higgins, C. A. Weatherford, and N. Salem, Jr. 2016. Global survey of the omega-3 fatty acids, docosahexaenoic acid and eicosapentaenoic acid in the blood stream of healthy adults. *Progress in Lipid Research* 63:132-152.

Stranaham, A. M., T. V. Arumugam, R. G. Cutler, K. Lee, J. M. Egan, and M. P. Mattson. 2008. Diabetes impairs hippocampal function through glucocorticoid-mediated effects on new and mature neurons. *Nature Neuroscience* 11(3):309-317.

Stranaham, A. M., K. Lee, B. Martin, S. Maudsley, E. Golden, R. G. Cutler, and M. P. Mattson. 2009. Voluntary exercise and caloric restriction enhance hippocampal dendritic spine density and BDNF levels in diabetic mice. *Hippocampus* 19(1):951-961.

Studenski, S. A., K. W. Peters, D. E. Alley, P. M. Cawthon, R. R. McLean, T. B. Harris, L. Ferrucci, J. M. Guralnik, M. S. Fragala, A. M. Kenny, D. P. Kiel, S. B. Kritchevsky, M. D. Shardell, T. T. Dam, and M. T. Vassileva. 2014. The FNIH Sarcopenia Project: Rationale, study description, conference recommendations, and final estimates. *Journals of Gerontology Series A: Biological Sciences and Medical Sciences* 69(5):547-558.

Susser, M., and Z. Stein. 1994. Timing in prenatal nutrition: A reprise of the Dutch Famine Study. *Nutrition Reviews* 52(3):84-94.

Tyrovolas, S., J. M. Haro, A. Mariolis, S. Piscopo, G. Valacchi, N. Tsakountakis, A. Zeimbekis, D. Tyrovola, V. Bountziouka, E. Gotsis, G. Metallinos, J. A. Tur, A. L. Matalas, C. Lionis, E. Polychronopoulos, and D. Panagiotakos. 2014. Successful aging, dietary habits and health status of elderly individuals: A k-dimensional approach within the multi-national MEDIS study. *Experimental Gerontology* 60:57-63.

UN (United Nations). 2015. *World population ageing 2015* (ST/ESA/SER. A/390). http://www.un.org/en/development/desa/population/publications/pdf/ageing/WPA2015_Report.pdf (accessed January 18, 2017).

USDA (U.S. Department of Agriculture). 2016. *Trends in food insecurity by race and ethnicity, 2001-15*. Economic Research Service. https://www.ers.usda.gov/data-products/food-security-in-the-united-states/interactive-chart-food-security-trends.aspx (accessed February 20, 2017).

USDA. 2017. *Healthy Eating Index*. Alexandria, VA: Center for Nutrition Policy and Promotion. https://www.cnpp.usda.gov/healthyeatingindex (accessed February 28, 2017).

Vos, M. B., J. L. Kaar, J. A. Welsh, L. V. Van Horn, D. I. Feig, C. A. Anderson, M. J. Patel, J. Cruz Munos, N. F. Krebs, S. A. Xanthakos, and R. K. Johnson. 2016. Added sugars and cardiovascular disease risk in children: A scientific statement from the American Heart Association. *Circulation* 135(3). http://circ.ahajournals.org/content/early/2016/08/22/CIR.0000000000000439 (accessed January 18, 2017).

Wall, T., K. Nasseh, and M. Vujicic. 2013. *Per-patient dental expenditure rising, driven by baby boomers*. Health Policy Institute Research Brief. Chicago, IL: American Dental Association. http://www.ada.org/~/media/ADA/Science%20and%20Research/HPI/Files/HPIBrief_0313_2.pdf?la=en (accessed January 3, 2016).

Wang, M., M. Li, S. Wu, C. B. Lebrilla, R. S. Chapkin, I. Ivanov, and S. M. Donovan. 2015. Fecal microbiota composition of breast-fed infants is correlated with human milk oligosaccharides consumed. *Journal of Pediatric Gastroenterology and Nutrition* 60(6):825-833.

Watabe-Rudolph, M., Y. Begus-Nahrmann, A. Lechel, H. Rolyan, M. O. Scheithauer, G. Rettinger, D. R. Thal, and K. L. Rudolph. 2011. Telomere shortening impairs regeneration of the olfactory epithelium in response to injury but not under homeostatic conditions. *PLOS ONE* 6(11):e27801.

Weaver, C. M., D. D. Alexander, C. J. Boushey, B. Dawson-Hughes, J. M. Lappe, M. S. LeBoff, S. Liu, A. C. Looker, T. C. Wallace, and D. D. Wang. 2016a. Calcium plus vitamin D supplementation and risk of fractures: An updated meta-analysis from the National Osteoporosis Foundation. *Osteoporosis International* 27(1):367-376.

Weaver, C. M., C. M. Gordon, K. F. Janz, H. J. Kalkwarf, J. M. Lappe, R. Lewis, M. O'Karma, T. C. Wallace, and B. S. Zemel. 2016b. The National Osteoporosis Foundation's position statement on peak bone mass development and lifestyle factors: A systematic review and implementation recommendations. *Osteoporosis International* 27(4):1281-1386.

Weindruch, R. H., and R. S. Sohal. 1997. Seminars in medicine of the Beth Israel Deaconess Medical Center. Caloric intake and aging. *New England Journal of Medicine* 337(14):986-994.

Weindruch, R. H., J. A. Kristie, K. E. Cheney, and R. L. Walford. 1979. Influence of controlled dietary restriction on immunologic function and aging. *Federation Proceedings* 38(6):2007-2016.

Weindruch, R. H., R. L. Walford, S. Fligiel, and D. Guthrie. 1986. The retardation of aging in mice by dietary restriction: Longevity, cancer, immunity and lifetime energy intake. *Journal of Nutrition* 116(4):641-654.

Westendorp, R. G. J. 2006. What is healthy aging in the 21st century? *American Journal of Clinical Nutrition* 83(2):404S-409S.

WHO (World Health Organization). 1948. *WHO definition of health*. http://apps.who.int/gb/bd/PDF/bd47/EN/constitution-en.pdf?ua=1 (accessed January 18, 2017).

Wojcicki, J. M., M. B. Heyman, D. Elwan, J. Lin, E. Blackburn, and E. Epel. 2016. Early exclusive breastfeeding is associated with longer telomeres in Latino preschool children. *American Journal of Clinical Nutrition* 104(2):397-405.

Wood, D., G. De Backer, O. Faergeman, I. Graham, G. Mancia, and K. Pyörälä. 1998. Prevention of coronary heart disease in clinical practice: Recommendations of the Second Joint Task Force of European and other Societies on Coronary Prevention. *Atherosclerosis* 140(2):199-270.

Wright, N. C., A. C. Looker, K. G. Saag, J. R. Curtis, E. S. Delzell, S. Randall, and B. Dawson-Hughes. 2014. The recent prevalence of osteoporosis and low bone mass in the United States based on bone mineral density at the femoral neck or lumbar spine. *Journal of Bone and Mineral Research* 29(11):2520-2526.

Wu, W.-K., S. Panyod, S., C.-T. Ho, C.-H., Kuo, M.-S. Wu, and L.-Y. Sheen. 2015. Dietary allicin reduces transformation of L-carnitine to TMAO through impact on gut microbiota. *Journal of Functional Foods* 15:408-417.

Yee, K. K., and N. E. Rawson. 2005. Immunolocalization of retinoic acid receptors in the mammalian olfactory system and the effects of olfactory denervation on receptor distribution. *Neuroscience* 131(3):733-743.

Zeevi, D., T. Korem, N. Zmora, D. Israeli, D. Rothschild, A. Weinberger, O. Ben-Yacov, D. Lador, T. Avnit-Sagi, M. Lotan-Pompan, J. Suez, J. Ali Mahdi, E. Matot, G. Malka, N. Kosower, M. Rein, G. Zilberman-Schapira, L. Dohnalová, M. Pevsner-Fischer, R. Bikovsky, Z. Halpern, E. Elinav, and E. Segal. 2015. Personalized nutrition by prediction of glycemic responses. *Cell* 163(5):1079-1094.

Zhu, S., K. V. Patel, S. Bandinelli, L. Ferrucci, and J. M. Guralnik. 2009. Predictors of interleukin-6 elevation in older adults. *Journal of American Geriatrics Society* 57(9):1672-1677.

Zhu, Y., and J. H. Hollis. 2015. Associations between the number of natural teeth and metabolic syndrome in adults. *Journal of Clinical Periodontology* 42(2):113-120.

Zonis, S., R. N. Pechnick, V. A. Ljubimov, M. Mahgerefteh, K. Wawrowsky, K. S. Michelsen, and V. Chesnokova. 2015. Chronic intestinal inflammation alters hippocampal neurogenesis. *Journal of Neuroinflammation* 12:65.

A

Workshop Agenda

Nutrition Across the Lifespan for Healthy Aging

Food Forum Workshop

September 13-14, 2016
National Academy of Sciences Building, Lecture Room
2101 Constitution Avenue, NW, Washington, DC

DAY 1, September 13, 9:00 AM-5:30 PM

9:00 AM **Welcome and Opening Remarks**
Sylvia Rowe, Food Forum Chair, SR Strategy, LLC, Washington, DC

9:05 AM **SESSION 1: Changing Landscape: Demographics, Health Status, and Nutritional Needs**
Session Moderator: Pamela Starke-Reed, Agricultural Research Service, U.S. Department of Agriculture

The Changing Face of Older Americans: Key Indicators of Well-Being
Jennifer Madans, National Center for Health Statistics
Healthy Aging Perspective
Mary Ann Johnson, University of Georgia
20-minute Discussion/Q&A

10:05 AM 25-MINUTE BREAK

10:30 AM **SESSION 2: The Spectrum of Aging and Health Over the Lifespan**
Session Moderator: Catherine Kwik-Uribe, Mars, Inc.

Early-Life Origins of Metabolic Disease and Aging
Janet King, Children's Hospital Oakland Research Institute
Biomarkers of Aging
Luigi Ferrucci, National Institute on Aging
Overweight and Obesity in Older Persons: Impact on Health and Mortality Outcomes
Gordon Jensen, University of Vermont Larner College of Medicine
30-minute Discussion/Q&A

12:00 PM **LUNCH BREAK (1 hour)**

1:00 PM **SESSION 3: Changes in Organ Systems Over the Lifespan**
Session Moderators:
Regina Tan, Food and Nutrition Service, U.S. Department of Agriculture
Sharon Ross, National Cancer Institute, National Institutes of Health

Selected Age-Associated Changes in the Cardiovascular System
Tamara Harris, National Institute on Aging
The Role of Nutrition on Cardiovascular Health and Disease in Aging
Penny Kris-Etherton, The Pennsylvania State University
15-minute Discussion/Q&A

Skeletal Systems
Connie Weaver, Purdue University
Muscular Systems
Roger A. Fielding, Jean Mayer U.S. Department of Agriculture Human Nutrition Research Center on Aging at Tufts University
15-minute Discussion/Q&A

3:00 PM **20-MINUTE BREAK**

Sensory and Oral Health
Age-Associated Changes in Taste and Smell Function
Nancy Rawson, Monell Chemical Senses Center
Nutrition and Oral Health in Aging
Athena Papas, Tufts University School of Dental Medicine
15-minute Discussion/Q&A

Early Nutrition, Gut Development, and the Microbiome
Nutrition and the Microbiome
Cindy Davis, Office of Dietary Supplements, National Institutes of Health
Noninvasive Methods for Assessing Nutritional Regulation of Neonatal Gut Gene Expression and Host–Microbe Interactions
Sharon Donovan, University of Illinois at Urbana-Champaign
15-minute Discussion/Q&A

Dietary Interventions for Healthy Aging
Rafael de Cabo, National Institute on Aging
10-minute Discussion/Q&A

5:30 PM **Adjourn Day 1**

DAY 2, September 14, 9:00 AM-12:00 PM

9:00 AM **Welcome and Opening Remarks**
Sylvia Rowe, Food Forum Chair, SR Strategy, LLC, Washington, DC

9:05 AM **SESSION 4: Moving Forward**
Session Moderator: Johanna Dwyer, National Institutes of Health and Tufts University

Nutrition to Promote Healthy Aging
David B. Reuben, David Geffen School of Medicine at the University of California, Los Angeles
10-minute Discussion/Q&A

What Are the Patterns of Dietary Intake Across the Lifespan and the Opportunities to Support Healthy Aging?
Eve Stoody, Center for Nutrition Policy and Promotion, U.S. Department of Agriculture
10-minute Discussion/Q&A

Supporting Healthy Aging Across the Lifespan: The Role of the Food Industry
Tim Morck, Spectrum Nutrition Consulting
Douglas "Duffy" MacKay, Council for Responsible Nutrition
15-minute Discussion/Q&A

MODERATED DISCUSSION
Moderator: Simin Meydani, Jean Mayer U.S. Department of Agriculture Human Nutrition Research Center on Aging at Tufts University

Healthy Aging: What Is It? Are There Acceptable Markers to Utilize in Developing Strategies to Promote It?
Panelists:
- Frank Busta, University of Minnesota
- Mary Ann Johnson, University of Georgia
- Janet King, Children's Hospital Oakland Research Institute
- David B. Reuben, David Geffen School of Medicine at the University of California, Los Angeles

12:00 PM ADJOURN WORKSHOP

B

Acronyms and Abbreviations

AI	Adequate Intake
ALM	appendicular lean body mass
BMD	bone mineral density
BMI	body mass index
CACFP	Child and Adult Care Food Program
CDC	U.S. Centers for Disease Control and Prevention
CNPP	Center for Nutrition Policy and Promotion
CRN	Council for Responsible Nutrition
DASH	Dietary Approaches to Stop Hypertension
DEXA	dual-energy X-ray absorptiometry
DGA	*Dietary Guidelines for Americans*
DGAC	Dietary Guidelines Advisory Committee
DHA	docosahexaenoic acid
DOHaD	International Society for Developmental Origins of Health and Disease
DRI	Dietary Reference Intake
EAR	Estimated Average Requirement
EPA	eicosapentaenoic acid
EPAS1	endothelial PAS Domain Protein 1

FDA	U.S. Food and Drug Administration
FITS	Feeding Infants and Toddlers Study
FNIH	Foundation for the National Institutes of Health
GI	gastrointestinal
GMA	Grocery Manufacturers Association
GSMAX	grip strength
$GSMAX_{BMI}$	grip strength adjusted for BMI
HAS	high-amylose starch
HDL	high-density lipoprotein
HEALTH ABC	Dynamics of Health, Aging, and Body Composition study
HEI	Healthy Eating Index
HHS	U.S. Department of Health and Human Services
HMO	human milk oligosaccharide
IGF-1	insulin-like growth factor-1
IHD	ischemic heart disease
IL	interleukin
IMT	intima-media thickness
LDL	low-density lipoprotein
MIND	Mediterranean-DASH Intervention for Neurogenerative Delay
MRC	Medical Research Council
NHANES	National Health and Nutrition Examination Survey
NIA	National Institute on Aging
NIH	National Institutes of Health
NOHS	Nutrition and Oral Health Study
NSS	Nutritional Status Survey
NT-proBNP	N-terminal pro brain natriuretic protein
ODS	Office of Dietary Supplements
OR	odds ratio
RCT	randomized controlled trial
RDA	Recommended Daily Allowance
RR	relative risk

SPRINT	Systolic Blood Pressure Intervention Trial
USDA	U.S. Department of Agriculture
USP	U.S. Pharmacopeial Convention
USPSTF	U.S. Preventive Services Task Force
WHO	World Health Organization
WIC	Special Supplemental Nutrition Program for Women, Infants, and Children

C

Speaker and Moderator Biosketches

Frank Busta, Ph.D., has been director emeritus of the National Center for Food Protection and Defense (NCFPD) since 2007 and professor emeritus of food microbiology at the University of Minnesota since 1999. Dr. Busta was named the first director of NCFPD in 2004, a position he held until 2014. Previously, he held faculty positions at the University of Minnesota, North Carolina State University, and the University of Florida. He served as chair of the Department of Food Science and Human Nutrition at the University of Florida from 1984 to 1987 and head of the Department of Food Science and Nutrition at the University of Minnesota from 1987 to 1997. Dr. Busta's research is in the areas of food safety, growth and survival of microorganisms in food after environmental stress, microbial ecology, and food defense. He has published more than 125 refereed research papers. Dr. Busta retired from the International Commission on the Microbiological Specifications for Food in 2002 after 15 years of service. He is a fellow of the Institute of Food Technologists, serving as its president in 1995-1996; the American Academy of Microbiology; the American Association for the Advancement of Science; the Institute of Food Science and Technology in the United Kingdom; the International Association for Food Protection; and the Academy of the International Union of Food Science and Technology. From 2011 to 2014, he chaired the Food Forum of the National Academies of Sciences, Engineering, and Medicine. Dr. Busta received his B.A. and M.S. from the University of Minnesota and his Ph.D. from the University of Illinois.

Cindy Davis, Ph.D., is director of grants and extramural activities in the Office of Dietary Supplements (ODS), National Institutes of Health (NIH). In this position, she actively engages and encourages partnerships with other NIH institutes and centers to facilitate funding of grants that are of high relevance to ODS's mission and goals. She is also actively involved in a number of government working groups on the microbiome. Before coming to ODS, Dr. Davis was a program director in the Nutritional Sciences Research Group at the National Cancer Institute (NCI). In 2000, she received a Presidential Early Career Award for Scientists and Engineers and was named U.S. Department of Agriculture Early Career Scientist. She has published more than 125 peer-reviewed journal articles and 11 invited book chapters. Dr. Davis received her B.S. in nutritional sciences with honors from Cornell University and her Ph.D. in nutrition with a minor in human cancer biology from the University of Wisconsin–Madison. She completed her postdoctoral training at the Laboratory of Experimental Carcinogenesis at NCI.

Rafael de Cabo, Ph.D., is senior investigator at the National Institutes of Health's National Institute on Aging; chief of the Translational Gerontology Branch; and chief of the Experimental Gerontology Section in the Aging, Metabolism, and Nutrition Unit. In 2004, he was appointed tenure track investigator in the Laboratory of Experimental Gerontology. Dr. de Cabo was tenured in 2009 and now heads the Experimental Gerontology Section (EGS). The EGS applies both physiological and tissue-specific molecular approaches to investigate effects of nutrition interventions on basic mechanisms of aging and age-related diseases. Its research is aimed at identifying protective mechanisms invoked by caloric restriction and evaluating the consequences of dietary interventions for lifespan, pathology, and behavioral function, and balances the exploration of in vivo rodent as well as in vitro paradigms of caloric restriction. Dr. de Cabo is editor-in-chief of the *Journal of Gerontology Biological Sciences*. He received his B.S. and M.S. from the University of Cordoba, Spain, and his Ph.D. from the Department of Foods and Nutrition, Purdue University. Upon completing his graduate education, he received a postdoctoral position in the Laboratory of Neurosciences at the National Institute on Aging.

Sharon M. Donovan, Ph.D., R.D., is Melissa M. Noel Endowed Chair in Nutrition and Health, professor, and interim director, Illinois Transdisciplinary Obesity Prevention Program, University of Illinois at Urbana-Champaign. She is actively involved in her professional societies, having served as 2011-2012 president of the American Society for Nutrition and currently serving as president-elect of the International Society of Research on Human Milk and Lactation (ISRHML). Her laboratory conducts basic and translational research in pediatric nutrition, currently focusing on optimizing the intestinal and cognitive development of neonates, development of the gut microbiome, and prevention of childhood obesity and picky eating in children. Dr. Donovan has published numerous peer-reviewed publications and book chapters and has garnered substantial research and training grant funding from governmental, private, and nonprofit organizations. She has received several awards in recognition of her research, including the Mead Johnson and Norman A. Kretchmer Awards from the American Society of Nutrition and the Erhlich-Kodovsky Young Investigator Award from ISRHML. She currently serves on the Food and Nutrition Board of the National Academies of Sciences, Engineering, and Medicine and the Food Advisory Committee of the U.S. Food and Drug Administration's Center for Food Safety and Applied Nutrition. Dr. Donovan received her B.S. and Ph.D. in nutrition from the University of California, Davis. She completed a postdoctoral fellowship in pediatric endocrinology at Stanford University School of Medicine, after which she accepted a faculty position at the University of Illinois at Urbana-Champaign.

Johanna Dwyer, D.Sc., R.D., is a senior nutrition scientist in the National Institutes of Health's Office of Dietary Supplements (ODS) and professor of medicine and community health at the Medical School and Friedman School of Nutrition Science and Policy, Tufts University. She is also senior scientist at the Jean Mayer U.S. Department of Agriculture Human Nutrition Research Center on Aging at Tufts University. At ODS her work involves the development of a Dietary Supplement Ingredient Database providing analytically substantiated values for key ingredients in dietary supplements, and the Dietary Supplement Label Database, a database of virtually all dietary supplements sold in the United States. Dr. Dwyer is involved in activities aimed at understanding motivations for and use of dietary supplements in Americans. She is the author or co-author of numerous publications on topics including preventing diet-related disease in children and adolescents, maximizing quality of life and health in the elderly, vegetarian and other alternative lifestyles, and dietary supplements. In addition to her work as a scholar and clinician, her interests in public nutrition policy have led to extensive involvement and assignments in Washington, DC. She was a member of the Food and Nutrition Board of the National Academies of Sciences, Engineering, and Medicine from 1990 to 2002 and has been active in a number of professional associations. Dr. Dwyer received her D.Sc. and M.Sc. from the Harvard School of Public Health and an M.S. from the University of Wisconsin, and completed her undergraduate degree with distinction at Cornell University. She is a member of the National Academy of Medicine and has served on its Council.

Luigi Ferrucci, M.D., Ph.D., is scientific director of the the National Institutes of Health's National Institute on Aging (NIA). He is a geriatrician and epidemiologist who conducts research on the causal pathways leading to progressive physical and cognitive decline in older persons. Dr. Ferrucci was named chief of NIA's Longitudinal Studies Section in 2002 and from 2002 to 2014 was director of the Baltimore Longitudinal Study on Aging. Between 1985 and 2002 he was chief of geriatric rehabilitation at the Department of Geriatric Medicine and director of the Laboratory of Clinical Epidemiology at the Italian National Institute of Aging. During the same period, he collaborated with the U.S. NIA. Dr. Ferrucci has made major contributions to the design of many aging-related epidemiological studies conducted in both the United States and Europe. He has redesigned the Baltimore Longitudinal Study on Aging to retain the wealth of data collected over more than 50 years while introducing new questions on the nature of aging that have emerged in the recent literature. Dr. Ferrucci received an M.D. and a Ph.D. in the biology and pathophysiology of aging at the University of Florence, Italy.

Roger A. Fielding, Ph.D., is director and senior scientist of the Nutrition, Exercise Physiology, and Sarcopenia Laboratory at the Jean Mayer U.S. Department of Agriculture Human Nutrition Research Center on Aging, Tufts University. He is also professor of nutrition at the Friedman School of Nutrition Science and Policy and professor of medicine at Tufts University School of Medicine. Currently, he serves as associate director of the Boston Claude D. Pepper Older Americans Independence Center. Dr. Fielding is an internationally known researcher who studies the underlying mechanisms contributing to the age-associated decline in skeletal muscle mass; the resultant impact on function; and the potential role of exercise, nutrition, and physical activity in attenuating this process. He has extensive experience in the conduct of randomized controlled trials of exercise, nutrition, and pharmacological therapies in older adults. Dr. Fielding has a strong record of extramural funding from both public- and private-sector organizations. He also serves as associate editor of the *Journal of Gerontology Medical Sciences* and of *Calcified Tissue International and Musculoskeletal Research*.

Tamara B. Harris, M.D., M.S., is senior investigator and chief of the Interdisciplinary Studies of Aging Section, Laboratory of Epidemiology and Population Sciences, National Institute on Aging (NIA). From Harvard, she joined the Office of Analysis and Epidemiology at the National Center for Health Statistics. She moved to NIA in 1991. Dr. Harris received her M.D. degree from Albert Einstein College of Medicine. She trained in internal medicine at Montefiore Hospital, Bronx, New York, and in geriatric medicine at Harvard University, Division on Aging, where she was a Kaiser

Fellow in Geriatric Medicine. She also obtained an M.S. in epidemiology from Harvard School of Public Health and has an M.S. in human nutrition from Columbia University College of Physicians and Surgeons.

Gordon L. Jensen, Ph.D., M.D., is senior associate dean for research and professor of medicine and nutrition at the University of Vermont Larner College of Medicine. His research interests focus largely on geriatric nutrition concerns. His team has emphasized the development and testing of nutrition screening and assessment tools in relation to specific functional and health care resource outcomes for older persons, with a particular focus on the impact of obesity on these outcomes. Dr. Jensen is past president of the American Society for Nutrition, past president of the American Society for Parenteral and Enteral Nutrition (ASPEN), and a current member of ASPEN's Foundation Board. He is also past chair of the Association of Nutrition Programs and Departments. He has served on advisory panels, study sections, or work groups for the National Institutes of Health, the American Dietetic Association, and the Food and Nutrition Board of the National Academies of Sciences, Engineering, and Medicine. Dr. Jensen received a Ph.D. in nutritional biochemistry from Cornell University and an M.D. from Cornell University Medical College.

Mary Ann Johnson, Ph.D., is Bill and June Flatt Professor in Foods and Nutrition at the College of Family and Consumer Sciences and interim director of the Institute of Gerontology at the College of Public Health, University of Georgia. She conducts research and outreach programs for older people to improve dietary habits, physical activity, and self-management of chronic diseases, and also studies centenarians. Through state and federal grants, Dr. Johnson and her staff provide nutrition, physical activity, wellness, and chronic disease self-management programs in communities. She serves on the board of directors of the Athens Community Council on Aging and also collaborates with faith-based organizations. She frequently speaks about aging, nutrition, and obesity at local, state, national, and international events. As part of the American Society for Nutrition's presidential line, Dr. Johnson will serve as the society's president in 2017-2018, previously having served the organization in several capacities. She is also a member of the Institute of Food Technologists and the Academy of Nutrition and Dietetics. Dr. Johnson received her B.A. in chemistry from the University of Northern Iowa and her Ph.D. in nutritional sciences from the University of Wisconsin–Madison.

Janet C. King, Ph.D., is a senior scientist at Children's Hospital Oakland Research Institute (CHORI). She also is a professor of nutrition at the University of California, Berkeley, and Davis. Dr. King is recognized internationally for her research in maternal nutrition and human zinc requirements. She has published more than 250 papers and trained more than 65 graduate students and postdoctoral fellows. She is the recipient of the International Underwood Award for Outstanding Research in Trace Elements, the W.O. Atwater award for distinguished nutrition research, and the Conrad Elvehjem award for public service in nutrition. She is a member of the National Academy of Medicine and the U.S. Department of Agriculture (USDA) Research Hall of Fame. Dr. King has been involved in implementing national and international nutrition policy throughout her career: she chaired the 2005 U.S. Dietary Guidelines Advisory Committee and initiated the Dietary Reference Intake process as chair of the Food and Nutrition Board of the National Academies of Sciences, Engineering, and Medicine. Prior to moving to CHORI in 2003, Dr. King directed the USDA Western Human Nutrition Research Center at the University of California, Davis (1995-2002), and chaired the Department of Nutritional Sciences, University of California, Berkeley (1988-1994), where she had served on the faculty since 1974.

Penny Kris-Etherton, Ph.D., R.D.N., is distinguished professor of nutrition in the Department of Nutritional Sciences at The Pennsylvania State University, where she has been on the faculty since 1979. Her research expertise is in cardiovascular nutrition. She conducts controlled clinical nutrition studies designed to evaluate the effects of nutrients, bioactives, and dietary patterns on risk factors for cardiovascular disease. Dr. Kris-Etherton has served on national committees in the United States that have issued dietary guidelines as well as guidelines for the control of blood cholesterol levels. Presently, she is vice-chair of the American Heart Association (AHA) Council on Lifestyle and Cardiometabolic Health and past chair of the AHA Nutrition Committee. Dr. Kris-Etherton is a fellow of AHA, the National Lipid Association (for which she served as president), and the American Society for Nutrition. She is the recipient of many awards in the field of nutrition and has published more than 330 papers in the peer-reviewed literature.

Catherine Kwik-Uribe, Ph.D., is global director of Applied Scientific Research and Scientific and Regulatory Affairs, Mars Symbioscience, a division of Mars, Inc., where she currently is responsible for managing scientific affairs and regulatory compliance. As part of her work at Mars, Dr. Kwik-Uribe has been actively involved in research on the unique role of bioactives in foods in supporting and optimizing health, with a particular focus on the bioactives in cocoa, known as cocoa flavanols. This global research program on cocoa flavanols has taken a multidisciplinary research approach to understanding the potential role of these compounds in supporting human health, with the research spanning from the development of validated analytical methods to human dietary invention trials. Dr. Kwik-Uribe also lends her expertise to Mars, Inc., on scientific issues related to human nutrition, health, and well-being. Since joining the company in 2002, she has remained actively engaged in research, having co-authored numerous papers and book chapters. Dr. Kwik-Uribe received her doctorate degree in human nutrition from the University of California, Davis, and was a postdoctoral fellow at the University of California, Santa Cruz, in the Department of Toxicology.

Douglas "Duffy" MacKay, N.D., is senior vice president, scientific and regulatory affairs for the Council for Responsible Nutrition, where he oversees the Science and Regulatory Affairs Department, ensuring that the association's scientific, policy, and legislative positions are based on credible scientific rationale. His expertise combines practical knowledge of industry regulation and scientific product development with hands-on experience as a medical practitioner. Dr. MacKay is a licensed naturopathic doctor who still sees patients on a part-time basis in an integrative medical practice; he previously was owner and practitioner in a complementary and alternative medicine private practice. He serves on the Advisory Board for the American Botanical Council, the National Science Foundation's International Joint Committee on Dietary Supplements, and the National Institute of Standards and Technology/National Institutes of Health Dietary Supplement Laboratory Quality Assurance Program. Dr. MacKay is also on the editorial board of three peer-reviewed publications: the official publication of the American Association of Naturopathic Physicians, *Natural Medicine Journal*; *Integrative Medicine*, a clinicians' journal; and *Current Topics in Nutraceutical Research*. He is also chair of the Steering Committee for the Standardized Information on Dietary Ingredients Work Group. Dr. MacKay earned his degree in marine biology from the University of California, Santa Cruz, and his N.D. from the National College of Natural Medicine in Portland, Oregon.

Jennifer H. Madans, Ph.D., is associate director for science at the National Center for Health Statistics (NCHS), where she is responsible for the overall plan for and development of data collection and analysis programs. Since joining NCHS, she has concentrated her research efforts on data collection methodology, measurement of health and functioning, and health services research. She has directed two national longitudinal studies, as well as the redesign of the National Health Interview Survey questionnaire. Dr. Madans was one of the designers of the U.S. Department of Health and Human Services' Survey Integration Plan. She is a founding member and chair of the steering committees for three initiatives aimed at developing internationally comparable measures of disability and health. She has also served as an adjunct associate professor in the Division of Biostatistics and Epidemiology, Department of Community and Family Medicine, Georgetown University School of Medicine, and in the Department of Demography at Georgetown. She is a fellow of the American Statistical Association and an elected member of the International Statistical Institute and served as a vice president of the International Association of Official Statistics. Dr. Madans received her B.A. from Bard College and her M.A. and Ph.D. from the University of Michigan. She completed a postdoctoral fellowship in the Department of Epidemiology and Public Health at Yale University.

Simin Nikbin Meydani, D.V.M., Ph.D., has served as director of the Jean Mayer U.S. Department of Agriculture Human Nutrition Research Center on Aging at Tufts University since 2009 and is currently transitioning to the position of vice provost for research at Tufts University. She is professor of nutrition and immunology at the Friedman School of Nutrition Science and Policy and the Tufts Sackler Graduate Program in Immunology. Dr. Meydani's scientific interests include the impact of nutrition on the aging process and age-associated diseases, the role of nutrition in immune and inflammatory responses, and predisposition to infectious diseases in developed and less developed countries. She is an internationally recognized scholar with more than 300 publications and has received numerous honors and awards. Her research is multidisciplinary and extends from cell and molecular to animal and clinical investigations. She has served as president of the American Society for Nutrition and the American Aging Association. She has also served the academic, government, and corporate communities as a member of a number of expert panels and boards, and has been a member of the editorial boards of several journals and chair of multiple summer conferences and other international meetings. Dr. Meydani holds a D.V.M. (Tehran University), an M.S. in nutrition (Colorado State University), and a Ph.D. in nutrition (Iowa State University).

Timothy A. Morck, Ph.D., is president and founder of Spectrum Nutrition LLC, a firm that provides expertise in nutrition-related basic/clinical research, product development, regulatory and public policy, and global scientific affairs. Dr. Morck's career includes clinical nutrition practice, research, and medical school faculty appointments; scientific association management; entrepreneurial personalized nutrition start-ups; and executive and senior management positions at several global nutrition and pharmaceutical companies. His unique multidisciplinary perspective integrates science and business objectives with a passion for personalized approaches to improving health. Dr. Morck received a B.S. in animal science from The Pennsylvania State University, followed by M.S. and Ph.D. degrees in nutrition (biochemistry and physiology minors) from Cornell University.

Athena Papas, D.M.D., Ph.D., is distinguished Erling Johansen professor of dental research and head of the Division of Oral Medicine at the Tufts University School of Dental Medicine. With expertise in the oral health care of the elderly and medically compromised, Sjögrens, cancer, and bone marrow transplant patients, Dr. Papas has been the principal investigator of more than 100 clinical trials. She co-authored a textbook titled *Nutrition in Clinical Dentistry*, and has conducted research on the interrelationship between nutrition and oral health in an aging population with the Tufts U.S. Department of Agriculture Human Nutrition Center on Aging. Dr. Papas was selected as the 2009 recipient of the International Association of Dental Research's Pharmacology/Therapeutics/Toxicology (PTT) Distinguished Scientist Award and has been the president of PTT. She has also received the Gavel and Pierre Fauchard awards and is a life fellow of the American College of Dentists. She received her dental degree from Harvard and her Ph.D. in oral biology from the Nutrition Department at Massachusetts Institute of Technology. She completed a predoctoral fellowship at Massachusetts General Hospital and a postdoctoral fellowship at Boston Children's Hospital.

Nancy Rawson, Ph.D., M.Sc., is associate director and associate member at the Monell Center, where she is responsible for managing corporate relationships and supporting strategy development and intellectual property management. As an associate member, she also conducts research in taste and olfactory cell biology. Dr. Rawson began her professional career as a nutritionist at Campbell Soup Company, providing nutrition guidance to product development and marketing teams and working with external researchers studying interactions between diet and health. She served as chief scientific officer at WellGen, Inc., directing research and development of therapeutic anti-inflammatory and antioxidant ingredients for the medical foods market. She then moved to AFB International, a global ingredient company serving the pet food industry, to build and lead the Basic Research and Innovation Teams. Dr. Rawson has held many advisory and teaching positions and has published more than 65 peer-reviewed research articles, reviews, and book chapters. She received her Ph.D. in biology at the University of Pennsylvania and holds an M.Sc. in nutrition from the University of Massachusetts and a B.Sc. from Fairfield University.

David B. Reuben, M.D., is director, Multicampus Program in Geriatrics Medicine and Gerontology, and chief, Division of Geriatrics, at the University of California, Los Angeles (UCLA), Center for Health Sciences. He is Archstone Foundation chair and professor at the David Geffen School of Medicine at UCLA and director of the UCLA Alzheimer's and Dementia Care program. Dr. Reuben is a past president of the American Geriatrics Society and former board chair, American Board of Internal Medicine. In

2012, he received one of the first Center for Medicare & Medicaid Innovation Innovation Challenge Awards to develop a model program for providing comprehensive, coordinated care for patients with Alzheimer's disease and other dementias. In 2014, Dr. Reuben was one of three principal investigators to be awarded a multicenter clinical trial by the Patient-Centered Outcomes Research Institute (PCORI) and the National Institute on Aging focused on reducing serious fall-related injuries—the largest grant PCORI has awarded. He also leads a grant aimed at determining and measuring patient and caregiver goals in Alzheimer's disease and dementia. In addition to his leadership in geriatrics, Dr. Reuben continues to provide primary care for frail older persons, including making house calls.

Sharon Ross, Ph.D., M.P.H., is a program director in the Nutritional Science Research Group, Division of Cancer Prevention, National Cancer Institute (NCI), National Institutes of Health. In this capacity, she is responsible for directing, coordinating, and managing a multidisciplinary research grant portfolio in diet, nutrition, and cancer prevention. Prior to joining NCI, Dr. Ross worked at the Center for Food Safety and Applied Nutrition, U.S. Food and Drug Administration (FDA), where she was involved in scientific review and regulation development for health claim labeling. Previously, she was a cancer prevention fellow in the Division of Cancer Prevention and Control, NCI. Dr. Ross holds a B.S. in nutrition and dietetics from the University of New Hampshire, an M.S. in nutritional sciences from the University of Connecticut, an M.P.H. from the Johns Hopkins Bloomberg School of Public Health with an emphasis in epidemiology, and a Ph.D. in nutritional sciences from the University of Maryland. She did her doctoral dissertation research in the Laboratory of Cellular Carcinogenesis and Tumor Promotion at NCI, focusing on the effects of retinoids in growth, differentiation, and cell adhesion.

Pamela Starke-Reed, Ph.D., is deputy administrator for nutrition, food safety, and quality at the U.S. Department of Agriculture's Agricultural Research Service (ARS). Prior to joining ARS in 2014, she was deputy director of the Division of Nutrition Research Coordination, National Institutes of Health (NIH), advising the NIH director and others on nutrition research issues and coordinating nutrition research and research training initiatives. Since 1991, she has served as adjunct professor with the George Washington University Medical Center. Dr. Starke-Reed is well known throughout the human nutrition community for her efforts at NIH to link research on nutritional sciences and physical activity to better understand how the quality of diet and physical activity contribute to health and disease/obesity. As part of that effort, she was co-chair of the Subcommittee on Dietary Reference Intakes of the Interagency Committee on Human Nutrition Research

(ICHNR), and she became co-executive secretary for ICHNR in 2014. She also serves on the editorial board of the *Journal of Nutritional Biochemistry* and as associate editor for *Nutrition Reviews*. She earned her B.S. in biology at St. Lawrence University and her Ph.D. in pathology at Hahnemann University.

Eve Stoody, Ph.D., is lead nutritionist of nutrition guidance for the Center for Nutrition Policy and Promotion (CNPP), U.S. Department of Agriculture (USDA). CNPP works to improve the health and well-being of Americans by developing and promoting dietary guidance that links scientific research to the nutrition needs of consumers. One of Dr. Stoody's primary assignments is to support the revision process for the *Dietary Guidelines for Americans*. She assisted the 2010 and 2015 Dietary Guidelines Advisory Committees throughout their deliberations, helped write the policy document for the 2010-2015 guidelines, and played a lead role in the development of the 2015-2020 guidelines. Dr. Stoody's team is also conducting foundational work to inform future dietary guidance for children from birth to 24 months and pregnant women. Prior to her current role at CNPP, she was a lead analyst for USDA's Nutrition Evidence Library, where she served as project manager for the Dietary Patterns Systematic Review Project. She was also a fellow at the U.S. Department of Health and Human Services Office of Disease Prevention and Health Promotion. Dr. Stoody received her B.S. in biology with a minor in nutrition from Texas Christian University and her Ph.D. in nutrition from Texas Woman's University.

Regina L. Tan, D.V.M., M.S., D.A.C.V.P.M., is director of the Office of Food Safety, Food and Nutrition Service, U.S. Department of Agriculture. She brings to this position more than 15 years of public health experience in preventive medicine, epidemiology, and systems analysis. Dr. Tan began her career as a Commissioned Corps officer in the U.S. Public Health Service and worked with the U.S. Centers for Disease Control and Prevention (CDC), first as an Epidemic Intelligence Service officer and then as a preventive medicine fellow. She joined the Food Safety Inspection Service (FSIS) as a veterinary epidemiologist in 2003. In 2005, she rejoined the CDC as a liaison with the Armed Forces Medical Intelligence Center, and in 2006 she joined The MITRE Corporation, where her management of a team of engineers was essential to developing innovative data architecture research and development across the federal government. She returned to FSIS in 2011 as director of the Applied Epidemiology Staff, and took over the Recall Management and Technical Analysis Division in 2013. Dr. Tan has led or served on numerous public health advisory committees, interagency teams, and working groups pertaining to threats to public health. She earned her D.V.M. and M.S. from Purdue University and her B.S. in biology from the

University of Maryland. She is also a Diplomate of the American College of Veterinary Preventive Medicine.

Connie Weaver, Ph.D., is distinguished professor and head of the Department of Nutrition Science at Purdue University. In 2015 she was appointed as a member to the U.S. Food and Drug Administration's Science Advisory Board. In 2014, she was appointed to the National Institutes of Health (NIH) Advisory Committee on Research on Women's Health. As founder and director of the Women's Global Health Institute at Purdue University, she oversees the mission of improving the health of women globally through research and training by proactively identifying the causes and prevention of diseases related to women. In 2008, Dr. Weaver became deputy director of the NIH-funded Indiana Clinical and Translational Science Institute. From 2000 to 2010, she was director of the NIH Purdue–University of Alabama–Birmingham Botanical Research Center, studying dietary supplements containing polyphenolics for age-related diseases. Dr. Weaver's research interests include mineral bioavailability, calcium metabolism, and bone health. She is past president of the American Society for Nutritional Sciences. She sits on several boards, has received multiple honors and awards, and has published numerous research articles. Dr. Weaver received a B.S. and an M.S. in food science and human nutrition from Oregon State University and a Ph.D. in food science and human nutrition from Florida State University. She is a member of the National Academy of Medicine and the Food and Nutrition Board of the National Academies of Sciences, Engineering, and Medicine.